Sexually Transmitted Diseases

Diseases and Disorders

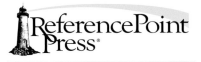

ReferencePoint
Press®

San Diego, CA

Other books in the Compact Research Diseases and Disorders set:

Anorexia
Anxiety Disorders
Bipolar Disorders
Bulimia
Depressive Disorders
Herpes
HPV
Influenza
Self-Injury Disorder

*For a complete list of titles please visit www.referencepointpress.com.

COMPACT *Research*

Sexually Transmitted Diseases

Peggy J. Parks

Diseases and Disorders

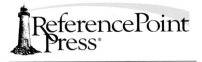

ReferencePoint Press®

San Diego, CA

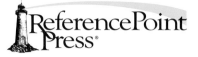

© 2014 ReferencePoint Press, Inc.
Printed in the United States

For more information, contact:
ReferencePoint Press, Inc.
PO Box 27779
San Diego, CA 92198
www.ReferencePointPress.com

Picture credits:
Cover: Dreamstime and iStockphoto.com
Maury Aaseng: 32–34, 46, 47, 59–61, 73–75
AP Images: 19
Science Photo Library: 14

LIBRARY OF CONGRESS CATALOGING-IN-PUBLICATION DATA

Parks, Peggy J., 1951- author.
  Sexually transmitted diseases / by Peggy J. Parks.
    pages cm. -- (Compact research series)
  Audience: Grade 9 to 12.
  Includes bibliographical references and index.
  ISBN-13: 978-1-60152-608-3 (hardback)
  ISBN-10: 1-60152-608-3 (hardback)
 1. Sexually transmitted diseases--Popular works. I. Title.
  RA644.V4.P375   2014
  616.95'1--dc23
                                                    2013033861

Contents

Foreword

As modern civilization continues to evolve, its ability to create, store, distribute, and access information expands exponentially. The explosion of information from all media continues to increase at a phenomenal rate. By 2020 some experts predict the worldwide information base will double every seventy-three days. While access to diverse sources of information and perspectives is paramount to any democratic society, information alone cannot help people gain knowledge and understanding. Information must be organized and presented clearly and succinctly in order to be understood. The challenge in the digital age becomes not the creation of information, but how best to sort, organize, enhance, and present information.

ReferencePoint Press developed the *Compact Research* series with this challenge of the information age in mind. More than any other subject area today, researching current issues can yield vast, diverse, and unqualified information that can be intimidating and overwhelming for even the most advanced and motivated researcher. The *Compact Research* series offers a compact, relevant, intelligent, and conveniently organized collection of information covering a variety of current topics ranging from illegal immigration and deforestation to diseases such as anorexia and meningitis.

The series focuses on three types of information: objective single-author narratives, opinion-based primary source quotations, and facts and statistics. The clearly written objective narratives provide context and reliable background information. Primary source quotes are carefully selected and cited, exposing the reader to differing points of view, and facts and statistics sections aid the reader in evaluating perspectives. Presenting these key types of information creates a richer, more balanced learning experience.

For better understanding and convenience, the series enhances information by organizing it into narrower topics and adding design features that make it easy for a reader to identify desired content. For example, in *Compact Research: Illegal Immigration*, a chapter covering the economic impact of illegal immigration has an objective narrative explaining the various ways the economy is impacted, a balanced section of numerous primary source quotes on the topic, followed by facts and full-color illustrations to encourage evaluation of contrasting perspectives.

The ancient Roman philosopher Lucius Annaeus Seneca wrote, "It is quality rather than quantity that matters." More than just a collection of content, the *Compact Research* series is simply committed to creating, finding, organizing, and presenting the most relevant and appropriate amount of information on a current topic in a user-friendly style that invites, intrigues, and fosters understanding.

STDs at a Glance

STDs Defined

Sexually transmitted diseases (STDs) include any infection or illness that can be spread through sexual contact.

Pathogens

STDs are caused by infectious organisms known as pathogens; these include bacteria, viruses, and parasites.

Types

Chlamydia, gonorrhea, and syphilis are bacterial STDs; human papillomavirus (HPV) and human immunodeficiency virus (HIV) are viral STDs; trichomoniasis and pubic lice are two common parasitic STDs.

Prevalence

According to the Centers for Disease Control and Prevention (CDC) there are more than 110 million cases of STDs in the United States, with about 20 million new cases reported each year.

STDs and Youth

The CDC states that adolescents and young adults aged fifteen to twenty-four account for nearly half of all new STD cases.

Symptoms

Depending on the STD, symptoms may include sores in the genital area; pain or burning during urination; abnormal discharge from the vagina or penis; rash anywhere on the body; fever; and/or abdominal pain.

STD Transmission

The most common way STDs are spread is through sexual intercourse (vaginal or anal) and oral sex; in some cases, they may be spread by fingers or other objects that have touched genitals or body fluids.

Dangers

If left untreated, STDs can lead to serious health problems, including organ damage, infertility, and possibly death; STDs in pregnant women can harm the fetus; the deadliest STD is HIV, which can advance to AIDS and destroy the immune system.

Diagnosis

A physical examination and a variety of tests (blood, urine, secretions from vagina or penis) can confirm the presence of an STD.

Treatment

Bacterial and parasitic STDs are easiest to treat because antibiotics can usually cure them; viral STDs are incurable but can often be managed with medications.

Prevention

The only sure way STDs can be avoided is by abstaining from any sexual contact; aside from that, risk can be lowered by consistent and correct use of latex condoms and limiting the number of sexual partners.

Progress in Fighting STDs

Medical research has broadened scientific knowledge and yielded numerous treatments so that many STDs can now be cured.

Overview

"Sexually transmitted infections are common in the United States, with a disproportionate burden among young adolescents and adults."

—Catherine Lindsey Satterwhite, a public health specialist and lead author of a major STD study published in March 2013.

"Sexually transmitted diseases (STDs) are an important global health priority because of their devastating impact on women and infants and their interrelationships with HIV/AIDS."

—National Institute of Allergy and Infectious Diseases, which conducts and supports research to better understand, treat, and ultimately prevent infectious, immunologic, and allergic diseases.

M ost people have some familiarity with warts, which are hard, bumpy growths that typically appear on the fingers, hands, toes, or soles of the feet. What is not so widely known is that warts can also develop in the genital areas of males and females, as the Centers for Disease Control and Prevention (CDC) explains: "They can be small or large, raised or flat, or shaped like a cauliflower." These are known as genital warts, and because they are spread through sexual contact, they are considered a sexually transmitted disease (STD). "Warts can appear within weeks or months after sexual contact with an infected partner," says the CDC, "even if the infected partner has no signs of genital warts."[1]

One young woman wrote about her personal experience with genital warts in a 2013 online article. Upon discovering the warts she was terribly distraught, as she writes: "I was on the toilet when I first felt the strange patches of raised skin. Because they weren't painful, the alarm took a moment to register. But when I got a closer look at the disturbance—bumpy white growths around the opening of my vagina—I immediately began to cry." The woman went to her gynecologist and was relieved when the doctor treated her with respect, rather than shaming or chastising her. Still, she felt "dirty and utterly tainted" for having caught the infection at all. "The stigma and shame of contracting an [STD] had done their job," she says. "At the moment of diagnosis, I felt like my life was over."[2]

How Pathogens Work

Genital warts are caused by the human papillomavirus (HPV), which is a family of viruses, including about forty types (strains) that can be sexually transmitted. Several other viruses can also cause STDs, as can some parasites and certain strains of bacteria. Learning about these pathogens (infectious organisms) is an important part of understanding what STDs are and how easily they are spread from person to person.

Bacteria are one-celled organisms that are relatively self-sufficient, meaning they have the capability of growing and multiplying on their own. They are often referred to as microorganisms because they are too tiny to be seen with the naked eye and are only visible through a microscope. "They're so small," says the Mayo Clinic, "that if you lined up a thousand of them end to end, they could fit across the end of a pencil eraser."[3] Most bacteria are not harmful to humans; in fact, many strains are beneficial, such as bacteria that live in the intestines and help keep the digestive system working properly. But pathogenic bacteria do exist. Once they attack human tissue they begin to grow and multiply rapidly and, in the process, damage and kill healthy cells.

> " **Viruses are even smaller than bacteria—up to one hundred times smaller.** "

Viruses are even smaller than bacteria—up to one hundred times smaller. An important way that they differ from bacteria is that viruses are incapable of multiplying on their own. Rather, they must invade and "hijack" the cells of plants or animals so they can replicate (make new copies of themselves) within those cells. "Otherwise," says infectious disease expert James M. Steckelberg, "they can't survive. When a virus enters your body, it invades some of your cells and takes over the cell machinery, redirecting it to produce the virus."[4] During this process host cells are destroyed, which allows toxins to spread throughout the infected person's body.

Parasites are described by the National Institutes of Health (NIH) as "very small animals that get nourishment from the person they infect."[5] Like viruses, parasites need a living host in order to survive, but they are even more dependent on the host than are viruses.

What Are STDs?

The simplest definition of an STD is any type of infection or illness that can be spread through sexual contact. Another term that is widely used is sexually transmitted infections (STIs), largely because "infections" has a broader meaning than "diseases." The American Sexual Health Association explains: "The concept of 'disease,' as in STD, suggests a clear medical problem, usually some obvious signs or symptoms. But several of the most common STDs have no signs or symptoms in the majority of persons infected. Or they have mild signs and symptoms that can be easily overlooked. So the sexually transmitted virus or bacteria can be described as creating 'infection,' which may or may not result in 'disease.'"[6]

The most common way STDs are spread is through vaginal, anal, or oral sex. It is possible, though, for certain pathogens to be spread by fingers or other objects that have touched genitals or body fluids. Contrary to popular myth, people cannot catch STDs through casual contact such as by shaking hands or sitting on a toilet seat. The Yale Medical Group writes: "STDs are not spread by handshakes, hugs, toilet seats, towels, dishes, telephone receivers, or insect bites."[7]

STD Prevalence

STDs are extremely common infectious diseases, as the American Congress of Obstetricians and Gynecologists writes: "Except for colds and flu, STDs are the most common contagious (easily spread) diseases in the United States, with millions of new cases of STDs each year."[8] The widespread prevalence of STDs has also been a consistent finding of the CDC. According to a CDC fact sheet published in February 2013, there are currently more than 110 million cases of STDs in the United States, with an estimated 20 million new cases reported each year.

Males and females of all ages, ethnicities, and walks of life contract STDs, as a University of North Carolina health services website explains: "The microbes that cause sexually transmitted diseases are equal opportunity bugs. They don't care if you are white or black, rich or poor, educated or illiterate, happy or sad. If you're a warm body, you'll do."[9] There are some age-related differences, however, as STDs are becoming increasingly more common among younger people. According to the CDC, although young people aged fifteen to twenty-four represent only 25 percent of the sexually experienced population, they contract nearly half of all new STDs.

Types of STDs

HPV is the most common viral STD as well as the most prevalent of all STD types. Herpes simplex is a viral STD as is human immunodeficiency virus (HIV). Although it is not as prevalent as many other STDs, HIV remains a significant threat. According to the CDC, nearly fifty thousand new cases of HIV are reported in the United States each year—and tens of thousands of people continue to be infected, as a March 2013 report by the Henry J. Kaiser Family Foundation explains: "While the number of new HIV infections (incidence) is down from its peak in the 1980s, new infections have remained at about 50,000 for more than a decade."[10]

The most common bacterial STD in the United States is chlamydia, followed by gonorrhea, and then syphilis. According to a 2013 CDC fact sheet, these three STDs account for nearly 2 million cases—yet their combined prevalence is not even half that of the STD known as trichomoniasis. It is caused by the *Trichomonas vaginalis* parasite, and leads to symptoms that range from mild irritation to severe inflammation. Another common parasitic STD is pubic lice, which are often called "crabs" because of their crab-like claws and body shape. About these organisms, the CDC writes: "Pubic lice usually are found in the genital area on pubic hair; but they may occasionally be found on other coarse body hair, such as hair on

> " The simplest definition of an STD is any type of infection or illness that can be spread through sexual contact. "

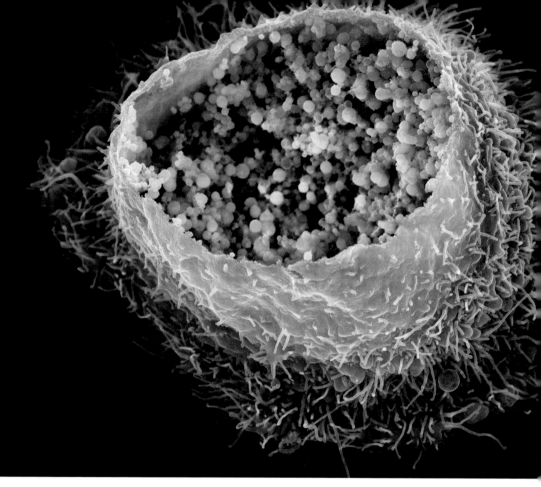

The most common bacterial STD in the United States is chlamydia, which can lead to infertility in women if not treated. Pictured is a scanning electron micrograph of a cervical cancer cell infected by chlamydia (small, round particles in the center).

the legs, armpits, mustache, beard, eyebrows, or eyelashes. . . . Lice found on the head generally are head lice, not pubic lice."[11]

Warning Signs

In many cases, people who have been infected by STDs are unaware of it because they do not develop any symptoms. When they do, symptoms can vary significantly depending on the particular STD and the health of the person who has contracted it. According to the Mayo Clinic, typical warning signs include sores or bumps in the genitals or rectal area; painful or burning urination; and discharge from the vagina or penis. Other possible symptoms include unusual vaginal bleeding; sore, swollen lymph nodes, particularly in the groin area; lower abdominal pain; and rash spread over the trunk, hands, and/or feet.

Syphilis is one STD that often escapes people's attention, at least at first, because its symptoms are easy to miss. In the early phase, an ulcer-like bump called a chancre (pronounced *shanker*) may develop at the location where the pathogen entered the body, such as the vagina, penis, mouth, or rectal area. "The sore is usually firm, round, and painless," says the CDC. "Because the sore is painless, it can easily go unnoticed."[12] If the disease is not treated, it progresses to what is known as the secondary phase. In addition to a new breakout of sores, symptoms may include fever, headache, and a rash anywhere on the body, such as the palms of hands and soles of the feet.

A seventeen-year-old girl named Amber caught syphilis from her boyfriend and says she first became suspicious after noticing "small, hard sores" in her vagina. "They didn't hurt," she says, "but when they didn't go away, I wondered if they came from having sex." Amber was dismayed to learn that her boyfriend had previously found similar bumps in his genital area. He had also suffered from ongoing fever as well as "strange dark red rashes on his hands."[13] Because his symptoms faded away, the young man did not realize that he was infected with syphilis and had unknowingly passed the disease on to Amber.

> " According to the CDC, although young people aged fifteen to twenty-four represent only 25 percent of the sexually experienced population, they contract nearly half of all new STDs. "

STD Risk Factors

Infectious disease experts stress that anyone who is sexually active can catch STDs. There are, however, a number of ways in which people put themselves at higher risk for becoming infected. Having unprotected sex is one of the biggest risk factors, as the Mayo Clinic writes: "Vaginal or anal penetration by an infected partner who is not wearing a latex condom transmits some diseases with particular efficiency. Without a condom, a man who has gonorrhea has a 70 to 80 percent chance of infecting his female partner in a single act of vaginal intercourse." Also at high risk are people with a history of STDs, as well as those who are sexually involved with multiple partners. "The more people you have sexual contact with," says the Mayo Clinic, "the greater your overall exposure risks. This is true for concurrent partners as well as monogamous consecutive relationships."[14]

> The most common bacterial STD in the United States is chlamydia, followed by gonorrhea, and then syphilis.

Sexually active people who drink alcohol or use illicit drugs have an especially high risk for contracting STDs. These substances are known to impair judgment and lower inhibitions—meaning those who get drunk or high are more likely to be careless about their sexual practices. "Drinking can make you take risks and do things you wouldn't normally do," says a young woman named Sara—who learned that lesson the hard way. In an online article published in July 2012, Sara speaks freely about the night that she got drunk and let "a handsome biker" take her home. Although she had never met the man before, she let him spend the night with her and had sex with him. "Now when I think about how risky it was," says Sara, "it makes me cringe."[15] Later, Sara "cringed" not only because of the risk she took, but also because of what resulted from the one-night stand: being infected with HPV and developing genital warts.

What Are the Dangers of STDs?

Innumerable health complications are associated with STDs, ranging in severity from skin rashes to cancer. "Each year," says infectious disease specialist Kimberly Workowski, "STDs cause at least 24,000 women in the U.S. to become infertile. Untreated syphilis can lead to serious long-term complications, including neurologic, cardiovascular, and organ damage." Workowski says that pregnant women who have syphilis can pass the disease along to the fetus, which can result in physical deformity, nervous system complications, and/or stillbirth. She adds: "Persons diagnosed with gonorrhea, chlamydia, herpes, or syphilis are at increased risk for HIV acquisition."[16]

Untreated chlamydia can be devastating to women, as the CDC explains: "Irreversible damage, including infertility, can occur 'silently' before a woman even recognizes a problem. Because symptoms of chlamydia are usually mild or absent, it can progress and damage a woman's reproductive organs and cause serious complications."[17] One of the most serious threats posed by chlamydia is pelvic inflammatory disease, which is a leading cause of infertility among women of childbearing age.

By far, the deadliest of all STDs is HIV because it destroys the immune system. The virus accomplishes its destruction by killing a specific type of white blood cell known as T lymphocyte cells, or T cells. These cells are crucial for fighting infection and disease. The National Institute of Child Health and Human Development (NICHD) writes: "Once HIV destroys a substantial proportion of these cells, the body's ability to fight off and recover from infections is compromised. This advanced stage of HIV infection is known as AIDS."[18] People with AIDS are extremely susceptible to opportunistic infections. These are illnesses that would pose a minimal threat for people whose immune systems are functioning properly; for those whose immune systems are damaged, however, the illnesses seize the "opportunity" to cause harm and can be deadly.

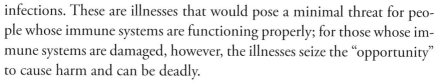

> One of the most serious risks posed by chlamydia is pelvic inflammatory disease, which is a leading cause of infertility among women of childbearing age.

Diagnosis of STDs

Depending on the type, STDs can often be diagnosed after a doctor performs a complete physical examination and takes a detailed sexual history. For both males and females, according to the NIH, the medical exam includes a thorough check of the genital area, oral cavity, and rectum. The group goes on to explain: "Many STDs can involve the mouth or rectum, especially when oral and anal sex are practiced. Swabs from open sores or discharges may be taken and tested for various microorganisms."[19]

To confirm whether someone has trichomoniasis, the physician views samples of vaginal fluid or secretions from the penis under a microscope. This is how the parasites can be identified, and according to adolescent medicine specialist Rima Himelstein, seeing the "wiggling organisms" is "an eerie sight." Whenever she finds that one of her young patients has developed trichomoniasis, she lets him or her take a look under the microscope to see what can result from having unprotected sex. She explains: "Seeing the infection can be the key to getting teens to change their risky behaviors—sometimes being spooked changes teens' behaviors."[20]

STD Treatment

In general, STDs caused by bacteria or parasites are easiest to treat because they respond so well to antibiotics. The Mayo Clinic writes: "Antibiotics, often in a single dose, can cure many sexually transmitted bacterial and parasitic infections, including gonorrhea, syphilis, chlamydia and trichomoniasis."[21] The group emphasizes the importance of patients following through with antibiotic treatment as well as abstaining from sex until the treatment program is complete and all sores have healed.

Viral STDs are not responsive to antibiotics and are not considered curable. Medical treatment is focused primarily on keeping symptoms under control, as the NICHD explains: "Health care providers can provide treatments to reduce the symptoms and the progression of most of these illnesses. For example, medications are available to limit the frequency and severity of genital herpes outbreaks while reducing the risk that the virus will be passed on to other people." The NICHD adds that people infected with HIV must take special medications known as antiretroviral drugs, which help control the amount of virus in their bodies. "These drugs . . . can help people live longer, healthier lives. If a woman with HIV becomes pregnant, these medicines also can reduce the chance that her fetus or infant will get the infection."[22]

How Can STDs Be Prevented?

"The only sure way to prevent sexually transmitted infections," says the CDC, "is to avoid having sex entirely."[23] In lieu of total abstinence, there are a number of precautions people can take to help reduce their

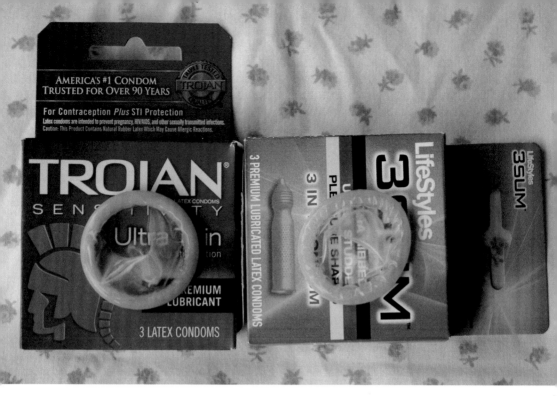

When used correctly and consistently, condoms can help prevent the transmission of STDs. But they do not entirely eliminate the risk of contracting an STD from an infected partner.

risk of STDs. These include avoiding sexual contact with those who are infected and having a mutually monogamous sexual relationship with someone who is known to be uninfected. Experts also emphasize the importance of limiting the number of sexual partners, since having sex with multiple partners is one of the biggest risk factors for STDs.

Another precautionary measure all sexually active people are strongly advised to take is using a latex condom correctly and consistently. Yet even condoms cannot offer 100 percent protection because they do not cover the entire genital area of either partner. These uncovered areas may be teeming with infectious viruses or parasites, and as a result the STDs can spread when the areas come into contact with unprotected skin.

What Progress Has Been Made in the Fight Against STDs?

Throughout the years, STD treatments have grown more sophisticated and effective, and this has made a significant difference in people's lives.

> **Viral STDs are not responsive to antibiotics and are not considered curable.**

Those with bacterial or parasitic STDs can often be cured with antibiotics. Although viral STDs are considered incurable, medical science has produced a number of drugs that help sufferers keep their conditions under control with few or no symptoms.

Especially profound is the progress made in the fight against AIDS. No longer is someone with HIV considered a lost cause—and that was the case not so long ago. Drugs known as antiretroviral medications can help HIV-positive people live healthy, happy lives without feeling as though death is imminent. Despite the progress, however, many challenges remain, and STDs are still considered a serious problem worldwide.

A Formidable Problem

STDs represent one of the biggest challenges faced by scientists and medical providers. These infections are extremely common and affect males and females of all ages and all walks of life. Many can be successfully treated and some can be cured, although STDs caused by viruses are especially challenging because the diseases are incurable. As research continues, new treatments will undoubtedly be discovered that help reduce the severity of STDs for those who suffer from them, which in turn will reduce the worldwide burden of these diseases.

What Are STDs?

> **66** STDs are among the most common infectious diseases in the world today. **99**
>
> —University of Maryland Medical Center, a teaching hospital in Baltimore that provides a full range of health services to people throughout Maryland and the mid-Atlantic region.

> **66** Sexually transmitted diseases (STDs) are occurring in high number among teenagers. **99**
>
> —American Academy of Pediatrics, which is dedicated to the health, safety, and well-being of infants, children, adolescents, and young adults.

I n early 1980 physicians in New York City and parts of Southern California began noticing a peculiar and disturbing trend: clusters of patients suffering from rare types of pneumonia and a rare form of cancer known as Kaposi's sarcoma. People with healthy immune systems did not typically develop these illnesses, so it was obvious that the sufferers had some type of immune system disorder. Adding to the mystery was that the patients were all gay men, as the Institute of Human Virology explains: "As such, many in the beginning of the early epidemic referred to the disease as GRID (gay-related immune deficiency). It was identified later as acquired immune deficiency syndrome (or AIDS) due to its nondiscriminatory, infectious spread around the world."[24]

By the beginning of July 1982 a total of 452 AIDS cases from twenty-three states had been reported to the CDC, and the casualties continued to climb. Health officials had no doubt that they were facing a public health crisis and something needed to be done—yet they had no idea what they were dealing with because the cause of the mysterious disease was still unknown. That changed in 1983 with an announcement by French scientists Françoise Barré-Sinoussi and Luc A. Montagnier. Working at the Pasteur Institute in Paris, France, they identified what later became known as human immunodeficiency virus (HIV), and they established a clear link between the virus and AIDS.

Then and Now

Although the discovery by Barré-Sinoussi and Montagnier was hailed as a major scientific accomplishment, questions lingered, particularly about the origins of HIV. It seemed to have appeared out of nowhere—where had it come from? Scientists offered a number of theories, but no one had any definitive answers until 1999, when that part of the puzzle was also solved. An international team of researchers announced that they had traced HIV's roots to a species of chimpanzee in western Africa. How the virus had made the jump from apes to humans was a matter of speculation, although the researchers had theories about it. They believed, according to the CDC, that the virus "most likely was transmitted to humans and mutated into HIV when humans hunted these chimpanzees for meat and came into contact with their infected blood. Over decades, the virus slowly spread across Africa and later into other parts of the world."[25]

> By the beginning of July 1982 a total of 452 AIDS cases from twenty-three states had been reported to the CDC, and the casualties continued to climb.

In the years since HIV's roots were discovered the number of Americans infected with the virus has grown, but new cases have gradually leveled off. The CDC estimates that 1,148,200 individuals thirteen years of age and older are currently living with HIV infection, and the annual number of new infections has remained at about fifty thousand cases per year. In 2011, for example, 49,273 people in the United States were diagnosed with HIV infection. This includes people of all ages, but of the newly reported cases, more than one-fourth were adolescents and young adults aged thirteen to twenty-four.

A young woman from California named Kelly never dreamed that she would be included in a statistic like that—but at the age of twenty-three she learned that she was HIV positive. This was a total shock, as she explains: "I wasn't having sex with multiple partners without condoms, wasn't sharing needles. I got infected by my boyfriend—who I trusted." Kelly remembers watching news programs about HIV and AIDS as a child, and she sometimes wondered how she would react to hearing such a diagnosis. "I remember thinking to myself, if I got diagnosed with HIV I would want to die," she says. "And then when it happened, it was a completely different reaction; it was no, this is not going to take over my life, I'm gonna get through this, this is not going to kill me." Yet she admits that coming to terms with the infection has been very difficult. "I have sat in my car and cried," she says, "and was screaming in the car with the windows rolled up. I have worked through those feelings."[26]

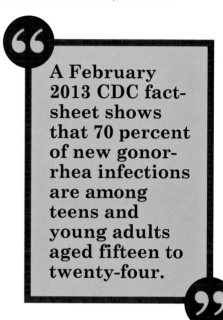

A February 2013 CDC factsheet shows that 70 percent of new gonorrhea infections are among teens and young adults aged fifteen to twenty-four.

Kelly says that "something really good that's come out of this" is that she has grown extremely close to her family and girlfriends and has a strong support system. But she is also a realist. "Don't get me wrong, HIV sucks," she says. "I don't want to admit I lost something, you know. I'm the one who's like, I'm gonna be positive no matter what, and I'm gonna tell you that everything is great and I'm getting through it . . . but in reality, I did lose a part of my youth."[27]

Young and Infected

In a March 2013 report called *Sexual Health of Adolescents and Young Adults in the United States*, the Kaiser Family Foundation covers a number of issues. One fact cited in the report is that despite education and prevention efforts, the incidence of STDs (also called sexually transmitted infections, or STIs) is higher among youth than older adults. "Sexually active teens and young adults are at higher risk for acquiring STIs," the authors write, "due to a combination of behavioral, biological, and cultural factors."[28] The authors go on to cite a CDC statistic about STDs and their growing prevalence among youth: that teens and young adults account for nearly 50 percent of new STD cases.

This statistic is based on averages, meaning that for some STDs young people account for a greater (or lesser) proportion. For example, a February 2013 CDC fact sheet shows that 70 percent of new gonorrhea infections are among teens and young adults aged fifteen to twenty-four. Another STD whose prevalence is high among youth is chlamydia, the most common bacterial STD in the United States. Of the 2.9 million new cases cited in the 2013 CDC fact sheet, 63 percent affected teens and young adults.

The "Silent" STD

According to Harry Fisch, a urologist from New York City, one reason chlamydia is so common is that it is a "silent" infection, meaning sufferers often have no symptoms. Thus, they are not aware that they have the disease and can spread it to sexual partners without knowing it. When symptoms do develop, women may have an abnormal vaginal discharge or a burning sensation when urinating. "If the infection spreads from the cervix to the fallopian tubes," says Fisch, "women may still have no signs or symptoms; others may have lower abdominal pain, low back pain, nausea, fever, pain during intercourse, or bleeding between menstrual periods."[29] Typical symptoms in men with chlamydia include a discharge from the penis, a burning sensation when urinating, and/or burning and itching around the opening of the penis.

> One reason chlamydia is so common is that it is a 'silent' infection, meaning sufferers often have no symptoms.

In 2011 health officials in Boston, Massachusetts, became aware of an unusually high rate of chlamydia in an area known as the Bowdoin-Geneva neighborhood. Community groups such as Big Sister Association of Greater Boston had noticed that the prevalence of chlamydia among Bowdoin-Geneva residents aged fifteen to twenty-four was nearly three times that of the city of Boston. Says Mia Roberts, a Big Sister vice-president: "Chlamydia is an issue in Bowdoin-Geneva—period."[30]

Roberts says that the problem was discovered while her group was working with the mayor's office to determine which community issues were most urgent and should be considered the highest priorities. They became alarmed when they saw the high number of youth who tested positive for the STD. "When we looked at the volume of data in Bowdoin-Geneva," says Roberts, "that's the one that jumped out at us."[31] City health officials do not know why chlamydia prevalence is so high.

The Dreaded Herpes

As common as chlamydia is, CDC data indicate that genital herpes is far more prevalent in terms of the number of people who are currently infected (new plus existing infections). According to the February 2013 CDC publication, more than 24 million people in the United States are living with genital herpes. Peter Leone, an infectious disease specialist at the University of North Carolina School of Medicine, says that most of those people do not know they are infected because they have no symptoms. "The classic description of genital herpes doesn't really match what we know in terms of the natural history normally," says Leone. "What I mean by that is if you pick up a textbook, you'll hear about all these painful ulcers and lesions, and you know, they last for days. The truth is that a minority of folks present that way."[32]

> **Although youth account for a large percentage of new STD cases, that does not mean that the infections are exclusively a product of being young.**

Herpes is caused by the herpes simplex virus (HSV). Leone says that there are "a bunch of different human herpes viruses,"[33] with the two primary types being HSV-1 and HSV-2. The former is usually associated with fever blisters or cold sores that develop on the lips, and for many years it was believed that only HSV-2 could infect the genital area. That is now known to be a false assumption, as Leone explains: "The idea . . . that HSV-2 is exclusively below the waist, and HSV-1 is exclusively above the waist causing cold sores is no longer true. So we really need to educate folks about what the differences are and why it's important to make the diagnosis to begin with." According to Leone, an increasing number of genital herpes cases are caused by oral sex. "What we're seeing is oral transmission that's primarily due to transmitting HSV-1 from mouth to genitals," he says. "So about 50 percent of the new genital herpes infections that we're seeing in the young adults now are due to HSV-1. And the clinical presentation for that is identical to HSV-2."[34]

No one needs to tell a young man named Victor that HSV-1 can cause genital herpes because, as he says, "I found out the hard way." When he was in college, Victor caught the virus by having oral sex and became aware of the infection when he developed painful symptoms. "I began to feel apprehensive when I felt as if I was urinating razor blades," he says. Although he hoped that he might have nothing more than a urinary tract infection or "some harmless condition that [would] go away with time," a doctor's visit confirmed his worst fears: genital herpes. "Learn from my mistake," he advises young people. "It could not, would not ever happen to me, except that it did."[35]

Not Just Kid Stuff

Although youth account for a large percentage of new STD cases, that does not mean that the infections are exclusively a product of being young. Studies have revealed some facts about STDs among older adults that are both startling and alarming to health officials. "Younger adults have far more STDs than older adults," says Massachusetts General Hospital researcher Anupam B. Jena, "but the rates are growing at far higher rates in older adults."[36] According to the CDC, there were 885 reported cases of syphilis among forty-five- to sixty-four-year-olds in 2000, and by 2010 the number had risen to more than 2,500. In that same time frame chlamydia cases among older adults soared, increasing from 6,700 in 2000 to more than 19,000 by 2010. HIV prevalence has also risen, nearly doubling among older adults since 2000.

Physicians and health officials have some theories about this rise in STDs among older age groups, one of which is lack of awareness. Prevention and education programs are targeted at youth, and those who are older often do not feel such precautions apply to them. Also, medications like Viagra are helping people be sexually active longer, while at the same time, studies have shown that older people are much less likely to use condoms than those who are younger. Florida physician Jason Salagubang shares his thoughts: "The flower children who were in their 20s back in the 1960s are now in their 70s. They're the make-love-not-war generation, and old habits die hard."[37]

Sexually Transmitted Misery

Scientists have learned a great deal about STDs over the years, and they continue to learn more through further studies. Yet even with all the knowledge and understanding that has been gained, millions of people of all ages continue to be infected every year. That is one unfortunate reality that physicians and health officials hope will change radically in the not-so-distant future.

Primary Source Quotes*

What Are STDs?

66 Many infections are sexually transmitted although some, including HIV and hepatitis B and C, are also transmitted by blood or blood products. **99**

—Lawrence R. Stanberry and Susan L. Rosenthal, *Sexually Transmitted Diseases: Vaccines, Prevention, and Control.* London, United Kingdom: Academic Press, 2013.

Stanberry is a professor in and chair of the Department of Pediatrics at Columbia University and New York–Presbyterian Morgan Stanley Children's Hospital, and Rosenthal is director of the Division of Child and Adolescent Health at the same facility.

66 Pubic lice (a.k.a. crabs) are nasty little parasites that require only brief contact to catch. . . . Oral sex has been shown to transmit crabs to eyelashes and eyebrows—not a pretty look. **99**

—Jake Deutsch, "Ask Dr. Jake: Can I Get STDs from Oral Sex?," *Daily Details* (blog), *Details,* February 8, 2013. www.details.com.

Deutsch is an emergency room physician in New York City.

Primary Source Quotes

❝We face a public health crisis of sexually transmitted diseases and unwanted pregnancies, in large part because so few people use condoms.❞

—Peter A. Ubel, "Why James Bond Needs to Use Condoms," *Psychology Today, Scientocracy* (blog), March 14, 2013. www.psychologytoday.com.

Ubel is a physician, behavioral scientist, and professor of business and public policy at Duke University.

❝STIs have been described since the beginning of recorded history in Europe and Asia, in handwritten manuscripts until the invention of the printing press by Gutenberg in 1454.❞

—Michael Waugh, "History of Sexually Transmitted Infections," in Gerd Gross and Stephen K. Tyring, eds., *Sexually Transmitted Infections and Sexually Transmitted Diseases*. London, UK: Springer Heidelberg Dordrecht, 2011.

Waugh is a physician in the United Kingdom.

❝There are many kinds of sexually transmitted diseases and infections. And they are very common—more than half of all of us will get one at some time in our lives.❞

—Planned Parenthood, "Sexually Transmitted Diseases (STDs)," 2013. www.plannedparenthood.org.

Planned Parenthood is the largest provider of reproductive health services in the United States.

❝STIs are very common in people under the age of 25.❞

—Palo Alto Medical Foundation, "Sexually Transmitted Infections (STIs)," 2013. www.pamf.org.

The Palo Alto Medical Foundation is a health care organization that serves the California counties of Alameda, San Mateo, Santa Clara, and Santa Cruz.

66STIs can affect men and women of all backgrounds and economic levels. However, some research suggests that STIs may be most prevalent among teenagers and young adults since they are more likely to have multiple sex partners during their lifetime.99

—Urology Care Foundation, "Sexually Transmitted Infections (STIs)," March 2013. www.urologyhealth.org.

The Urology Care Foundation promotes research and education in the field of urology, the branch of medicine related to the urinary system.

66Many STDs cause no symptoms in some people, which is one of the reasons experts prefer the term 'sexually transmitted infections' to 'sexually transmitted diseases.'99

—Mayo Clinic, "Sexually Transmitted Diseases (STDs)," February 23, 2013. www.mayoclinic.com.

The Mayo Clinic is a world-renowned health care facility that is dedicated to patient care, education, and research.

66Despite the fact that STDs are extremely widespread, most people in the United States remain unaware of the risk and consequences of all but the most prominent STD—HIV, the virus that causes AIDS.99

—Centers for Disease Control and Prevention (CDC), "STDs Today," National Prevention Information Network, April 16, 2013. www.cdcnpin.org.

The CDC is the United States' leading health protection agency.

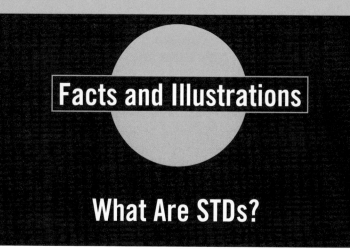

Facts and Illustrations

What Are STDs?

- According to a February 2013 CDC fact sheet, there are nearly **20 million** new STD infections each year in the United States, with more than half affecting young people aged fifteen to twenty-four.

- The Foundation for AIDS research says that at least two teenagers and young adults in the United States are infected with HIV **every hour of every day**.

- According to the National Institute of Allergy and Infectious Diseases (NIAID), about **two-thirds** of people who have sexual contact with a partner with **genital warts** will develop the infection, usually within three months of contact.

- The World Health Organization states that in developing countries, STDs and their complications rank in the **top five** disease categories for which adults seek health care.

- In July 2011 infectious disease expert Charlotte Gaydos announced a study of 7,593 American women aged 18 to 89 that found women 50 and older had the highest rate of trichomoniasis (**13 percent**) followed by women in their forties s at **11 percent**.

- According to University of North Carolina infectious disease specialist Christopher Hurt, studies of patients visiting STD clinics have revealed that **5 to 10 percent** have gonorrhea of the throat, which was contracted through oral sex.

HPV Outnumbers All Other STDs

A February 2013 report on STDs by the Centers for Disease Control and Prevention shows that there are more than 110 million cases nationwide in the United States. As this graph shows, the human papillomavirus (HPV) is far more common than all other types of STDs.

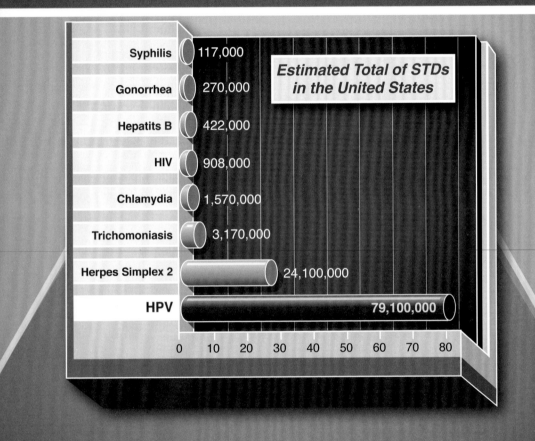

Estimated Total of STDs in the United States

Syphilis	117,000
Gonorrhea	270,000
Hepatits B	422,000
HIV	908,000
Chlamydia	1,570,000
Trichomoniasis	3,170,000
Herpes Simplex 2	24,100,000
HPV	79,100,000

Source: Centers for Disease Control and Prevention, "Incidence, Prevalence, and Cost of Sexually Transmitted Infections in the United States," CDC Fact Sheet, February 2013. www.cdc.gov.

- Infectious disease specialist Kimberly Workowski states that between 2005 and 2009 syphilis rates increased **167 percent** among black men aged 15 to 19 and **212 percent** among black men aged 20 to 24.

High HIV-Infection Rates in Africa

A report published in December 2012 by an Australia-based research group shows that three African countries—Zambia, Zimbabwe, and South Africa—have much higher rates of HIV infection than other countries.

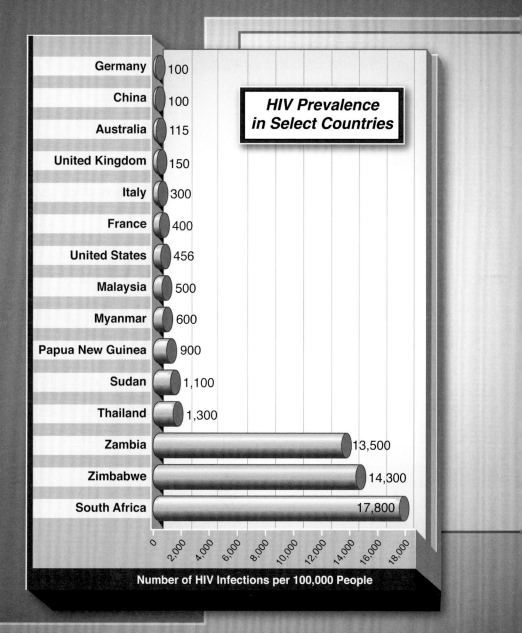

HIV Prevalence in Select Countries

Country	Number of HIV Infections per 100,000 People
Germany	100
China	100
Australia	115
United Kingdom	150
Italy	300
France	400
United States	456
Malaysia	500
Myanmar	600
Papua New Guinea	900
Sudan	1,100
Thailand	1,300
Zambia	13,500
Zimbabwe	14,300
South Africa	17,800

Number of HIV Infections per 100,000 People

Source: Kirby Institute for Infection and Immunity in Society, "HIV, Viral Hepatitis, and Sexually Transmissible Infections in Australia: Annual Surveillance Report 2012," December 5, 2012. www.kirby.unsw.edu.au.

Chlamydia and Gonorrhea Highest Among African Americans

STDs affect males and females of all ages, ethnicities, and walks of life. But in the United States, as this graph illustrates, chlamydia and gonorrhea are significantly more common among African Americans than Hispanics and Caucasians.

New Chlamydia and Gonorrhea Infections (2011) by Race/Ethnicity

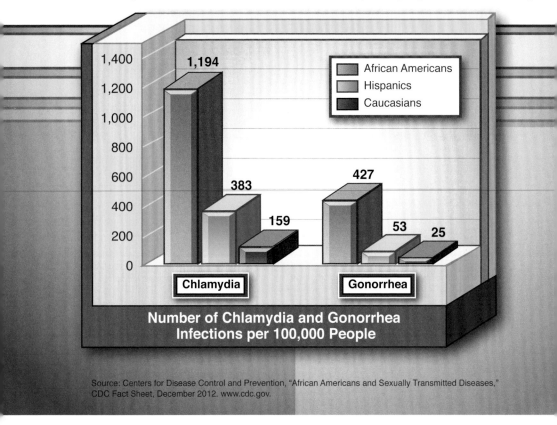

Source: Centers for Disease Control and Prevention, "African Americans and Sexually Transmitted Diseases," CDC Fact Sheet, December 2012. www.cdc.gov.

- According to a February 2013 fact sheet by the CDC, **20 percent** of people with HPV are infected with more than one type of the virus.

- The Urology Care Foundation estimates that there are from **4 million to 8 million** new cases of chlamydia every year.

What Are the Dangers of STDs?

66 Sexually transmitted infections (STIs) are a major global cause of acute illness, infertility, long-term disability, and death, with serious medical and psychological consequences. 99

—World Health Organization, the directing and coordinating authority for health within the United Nations system.

66 STIs . . . can be relatively harmless or they can be painful, irritating, debilitating and even life threatening. 99

—Urology Care Foundation, which promotes research and education in the field of urology, the branch of medicine related to the urinary system.

Jessica, a young woman from the United Kingdom, was twenty years old when she received heartbreaking news from her doctor: Because of damage to her reproductive system, she would probably never be able to have children. In an October 2011 article, Jessica says her nightmare began when she developed severe abdominal pain, which she assumed was related to her menstrual cycle. When the pain continued to get worse Jessica went to a clinic for an examination and was shocked to learn that she had chlamydia. She later discovered she got it from her former boyfriend, who had contracted it from another woman. Jessica had no idea he had infected her because more than a year went by before she had any symptoms.

After being diagnosed, Jessica was given antibiotics for the chlamydia and sent to a hospital for testing because of her abdominal pain. During exploratory surgery doctors discovered thick scar tissue in both of her fallopian tubes, which are the slender ducts that carry eggs from the ovaries to the uterus. This had resulted from pelvic inflammatory disease (PID), a severe infection of the genital tract that had developed when Jessica's chlamydia remained untreated. The scarring is so severe that Jessica has no more than a 10 percent chance of being able to get pregnant. "I'm devastated," she says. "I've been given a slim chance I'll ever have children. I'm so young, but I don't feel young anymore. I feel old and useless. . . . I've been torn into pieces by this."[38]

Severe Complications

PID is one of the most serious threats posed by untreated chlamydia, as well as gonorrhea. It develops when bacteria in the vagina spread upward and into the reproductive organs, including the uterus, cervix, ovaries, and fallopian tubes. As was the case with Jessica, infection in the fallopian tubes can lead to severe scarring. "Infection-causing bacteria can silently invade the fallopian tubes," says the CDC, "causing normal tissue to turn into scar tissue. This scar tissue blocks or interrupts the normal movement of eggs into the uterus." The CDC goes on to explain how this can lead to infertility: "If the fallopian tubes are totally blocked by scar tissue, sperm cannot fertilize an egg, and the woman becomes infertile. Infertility also can occur if the fallopian tubes are partially blocked or even slightly damaged."[39]

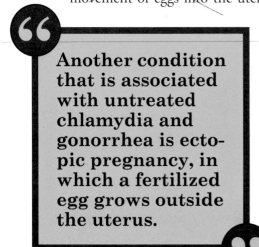

Another condition that is associated with untreated chlamydia and gonorrhea is ectopic pregnancy, in which a fertilized egg grows outside the uterus.

Along with PID, another condition that is associated with untreated chlamydia and gonorrhea is ectopic pregnancy, in which a fertilized egg grows outside the uterus. This often happens in a fallopian tube that has become blocked or slightly damaged, and is a potentially life-threatening condition. The CDC explains: "As it grows, an ectopic pregnancy can rupture the fallopian tube causing severe pain, internal bleeding, and even death."[40]

A study published in January 2011 by researchers from Edinburgh University in Scotland focused on the connection between chlamydia and ectopic pregnancy. The team found that women who had the STD were more likely to produce a protein in their fallopian tubes called PROKR2, and that increased the likelihood of an embryo becoming implanted in one of the tubes. Says lead researcher Andrew Horne: "We know that chlamydia is a major risk factor for ectopic pregnancy but until now we were unsure how

> **Untreated trichomoniasis can also be dangerous for men because it has been linked to cancer of the prostate.**

the infection led to implantation of a pregnancy in the Fallopian tube. We hope that this new information allows health care providers to give women accurate information about risks following chlamydial infection and to support public health messages about the importance of safer sex and chlamydia testing."[41]

Perilous Parasites

One of the most common STDs is trichomoniasis, which is caused by the single-celled parasite *Trichomonas vaginalis*. Infectious disease specialists say that about 70 percent of those who are infected by the parasite are unaware of it either because they have no symptoms or because they do not recognize the symptoms; thus, they do not seek treatment. In women, this can lead to inflammation of the vagina, urethra (the tube that carries urine away from the bladder and out of the body), and cervix, as well as to the development of PID. In pregnant women, untreated trichomoniasis has been associated with premature labor and low-birth-weight babies.

Untreated trichomoniasis can also be dangerous for men because it has been linked to cancer of the prostate, which is the small gland that surrounds the urethra. Scientists have long suspected that prostate cancer could be linked to one or more STDs but could not find any connections with chlamydia, gonorrhea, HIV, HPV, or herpes. Research done by scientists at Washington State University suggests that trichomoniasis is the link. Researcher John Alderete says that the *Trichomonas* parasite activates a group of proteins, one of which ensures that the proteins stay active. "It's like switching a light switch on," he says. "Then, if you don't control the brightness of that light, you can go blind. That's the problem."[42] Alderete goes on to say that men who suffer from trichomoniasis and are not treated have a 40 percent greater chance of developing prostate cancer than the general male population.

A study published in the September 2009 issue of the *Journal of the National Cancer Institute* also focused on the connection between trichomoniasis and prostate cancer. Conducted by a team of researchers from the Harvard School of Public Health, the study involved analysis of blood samples from 673 men with prostate cancer and a control group of 673 healthy men. The researchers compared the blood samples and recorded their findings.

> **By far, the most common form of HPV-associated cancer is cervical cancer, which affects more than twelve thousand women each year.**

They discovered that roughly one out of five men had been infected by the *Trichomonas* parasite at some point during their lives. Those with prostate cancer who had the STD in the past were two to three times more likely to develop an aggressive and potentially life-threatening form of the cancer. University of Connecticut prostate cancer researcher Peter C. Albertsen, who was not part of the Harvard study but wrote an accompanying editorial, shares his thoughts: "What this study explores and similar studies are exploring is whether there are potentially infectious causes that result in prostate cancer going from a relatively dormant disease to one that's clinically significant. This study raises the issue that a common bug, *Trichomonas vaginalis*, could be such an agent."[43]

The Cancer Virus

Of more than one hundred types of HPV that have been identified by scientists, about forty can infect the genital areas of males and females. Some of these, known as high-risk or oncogenic HPVs, are known to cause cancer. Among men, the CDC says that HPV causes an estimated 1,500 anal cancers and 600 penile cancers each year. In women, HPV causes approximately 2,800 cancers of the anus, 2,100 cancers of the vulva, and 500 cancers of the vagina. By far, the most common form of

HPV-associated cancer is cervical cancer, which affects more than twelve thousand women each year. The National Cancer Institute writes: "Virtually all cervical cancers are caused by HPV infections, with just two HPV types, 16 and 18, responsible for about 70 percent of all cases."[44]

Rose Hansen was only twenty-two years old when she was diagnosed with cervical cancer. Unlike many women who have no symptoms, Hansen had developed abnormal bleeding, as she writes: "It first appeared as small red butterflies that stained the sheets, ink blots on my underwear. Every time after sex, I bled; thin rivulets that trickled down my legs, begging to be deciphered."[45] Most everyone she talked to said the bleeding was "probably nothing,"[46] including her boyfriend, the nurse at the doctor's office, and even the doctor herself. Still, Hansen had a nagging feeling that the bleeding was indeed something to worry about—and she proved to be correct.

> **Although HPV is most commonly spread through sexual intercourse, research has clearly shown that some high-risk strains can also be spread through oral sex.**

After a test, the doctor called with a lengthy, complicated-sounding name for Hansen's condition: high-grade squamous intraepithelial lesion indicative of moderate to severe neoplasia or carcinoma in situ (HSIL). "I had no idea what that meant," says Hansen, "but carcinoma, which I knew meant cancer, leaped at me with claws. My heart stomped in my ears. . . . Afterward, I called my boyfriend, recited 'HSIL' and 'carcinoma in situ,' carcinoma, carcinoma, carcinoma thundering beneath my scalp."[47] Hansen underwent a surgical procedure to have the cancerous tissue removed. Five months later she had follow-up tests and was distraught when they showed that some cancer remained—and it was more aggressive and faster-growing than is typical. She underwent another procedure and the doctor said she had gotten it all, but there was no guarantee that it would not flare up again. "It might come back," says Hansen. "Always I am haunted by this."[48]

Risky Oral Sex

Although HPV is most commonly spread through sexual intercourse, research has clearly shown that some high-risk strains can also be spread through oral sex. This can lead to oropharyngeal cancers, in which malignant (cancerous) cells form in the tissues of the tongue, soft palate, tonsils, and side and back walls of the throat. The CDC estimates that each year seventeen hundred oropharyngeal cancers are diagnosed in women and seven thousand cases are diagnosed in men. According to a study published in the *Journal of Clinical Oncology* in November 2011, oropharyngeal cancer prevalence "increased substantially" from 16.3 percent during the 1980s to nearly 73 percent in 2004. The study authors say that this increase "perhaps arises from increased oral sex and oral HPV exposure over calendar time."[49]

In June 2013 actor Michael Douglas had a candid interview with a reporter from the British newspaper *Guardian*. Douglas had previously announced that he was being treated for throat cancer. Not until the 2013 interview, however, did he reveal that the cancer was caused by HPV and that he had caught it from performing oral sex on women. Currently in remission, Douglas spoke about feeling happy and grateful, as he explains: "It's been a rough few years, the cancer break. But I'm back with a vengeance. I feel blessed and fortunate that I still have a career. I feel blessed and fortunate that I'm even alive."[50]

The Deadliest Virus

Of all the STDs that are known to exist, HIV is the most feared. The virus is particularly deadly because it attacks and destroys the body's immune system—the very thing that is supposed to *keep* people from getting sick. Composed of a network of white blood cells (leukocytes), tissues, and organs that work together harmoniously, the immune system acts as the first line of defense against infectious organisms and other invaders. Children's Hospital Colorado writes: "Through a series of steps called the immune response, the immune system attacks organisms and substances that invade body systems and cause disease."[51]

Ordinarily, the immune system has the ability to seek out and kill viruses fairly quickly, such as when someone has a stomach virus or cold and recovers after a period of time. HIV, however, is a different kind of virus—one that zeroes in on the immune system itself. HIV accomplishes this by finding and destroying one specific type of immune system cell known as a CD4 lymphocyte. The patient advocacy group Global Fund writes: "HIV has a number of tricks that help it to evade the body's defenses, including very rapid mutation. This means that once HIV has taken hold, the immune system can never fully get rid of it."[52]

Once HIV has damaged someone's immune system, that system is not only more vulnerable to the virus but also to the attacks of other infections. The immune system "won't always have the strength to fight off things that wouldn't have bothered it before," says the Global Fund. As time goes by, an individual who has an HIV infection will likely become sick more and more often until he or she becomes ill with one or more severe illnesses. This is the phase where the infected person is said to have AIDS, as the group writes: "AIDS is an extremely serious condition, and at this stage the body has very little defense against any sort of infection."[53]

A Multitude of Dangers

From pelvic inflammatory disease and ectopic pregnancy to cancer and AIDS, the risks posed by STDs are numerous. For people who discover that they are infected, treatment can help avoid most life-threatening problems. But because many of these infections are asymptomatic, they often go unnoticed—and in the process, they can cause irreparable damage.

What Are the Dangers of STDs?

66 **While HIV is certainly dangerous, and even thinking about it can be scary, it's not the only STD that can be dangerous for teens to obtain.** 99

—Newport Academy, "Sexually Transmitted Diseases," 2013. www.newportacademy.com.

Newport Academy is a Southern California teen treatment center.

....

66 **Sexually transmitted diseases can cause severe damage to your body—even death.** 99

—American Congress of Obstetricians and Gynecologists (ACOG), "How to Prevent Sexually Transmitted Diseases," May 2011. www.acog.org.

Composed of approximately fifty-five thousand physician members, the ACOG is the United States' leading advocate for women's quality health care.

....

* Editor's Note: While the definition of a primary source can be narrowly or broadly defined, for the purposes of Compact Research, a primary source consists of: 1) results of original research presented by an organization or researcher; 2) eyewitness accounts of events, personal experience, or work experience; 3) first-person editorials offering pundits' opinions; 4) government officials presenting political plans and/or policies; 5) representatives of organizations presenting testimony or policy.

❝STIs in infants can cause serious problems and may be fatal.❞

—Mayo Clinic, "Sexually Transmitted Diseases (STDs)," February 23, 2013. www.mayoclinic.com.

The Mayo Clinic is a world-renowned health care facility that is dedicated to patient care, education, and research.

❝Infection with certain STDs can increase the risk of getting and transmitting HIV as well as alter the way the disease progresses. In addition, STDs can cause long-term health problems.❞

—National Institute of Allergy and Infectious Diseases (NIAID), "Sexually Transmitted Diseases (STDs)," July 15, 2011. www.niaid.nih.gov.

The NIAID conducts and supports research to better understand, treat, and ultimately prevent infectious, immunologic, and allergic diseases.

❝Because symptoms of chlamydia are usually mild or absent, it can progress and damage a woman's reproductive organs and cause serious complications.❞

—Centers for Disease Control and Prevention (CDC), "STDs Today," National Prevention Information Network, April 16, 2013. www.cdcnpin.org.

The CDC is the United States' leading health protection agency.

❝Gonorrhea also can infect the mouth, throat, eyes, and rectum and can spread to the blood and joints, where it can become a life-threatening illness.❞

—National Institute of Child Health and Human Development (NICHD), "What Are Some Types of STDs/STIs?," November 30, 2012. www.nichd.nih.gov.

The NICHD conducts and supports laboratory research, clinical trials, and epidemiological studies.

66 Most STDs affect both men and women, but in many cases the health problems they cause can be more severe for women. **99**

—National Institutes of Health, "Sexually Transmitted Diseases," July 16, 2013. www.nlm.nih.gov.

The National Institutes of Health is the United States' primary scientific research agency and the largest source of medical research funding in the world.

66 A variety of cancers can be caused by particular sexually transmitted infections. **99**

—Planned Parenthood, "Sexually Transmitted Infections Q & A," 2013. www.plannedparenthood.org.

Planned Parenthood is the largest provider of reproductive health services in the United States.

Facts and Illustrations

What Are the Dangers of STDs?

- According to the CDC, in the late stages of syphilis the disease damages internal organs including the brain, nerves, eyes, heart, blood vessels, and liver, and can **result in death**.

- The NICHD states that if gonorrhea is not treated it can spread to the blood and joints, where it becomes a **life-threatening** illness.

- According to a 2011 study led by National Cancer Institute researcher Anil K. Chaturvedi, if incidence trends continue, the annual number of **HPV-positive throat cancers** is expected to surpass the annual number of cervical cancers by the year 2020.

- Infectious disease specialist Kimberly Workowski states that each year STDs cause at least **24,000** women in the United States to become infertile.

- A spring 2013 article in a publication by Johns Hopkins Medicine states that one type of HPV (HPV 16) alone accounts for **50 percent** of all cervical cancers and most head and neck cancers.

- According to the CDC, from **10 to 15 percent** of women with pelvic inflammatory disease become infertile.

- The NIH states that during later stages of AIDS, pneumonia or cancer may develop, which can ultimately **lead to death**.

STDs Carry Serious Health Risks

The severity of health risks associated with STDs depends on the type of STD and how long the patient goes without treatment. This diagram illustrates the potential effects of some of the most common and familiar STDs.

STD	Potential Health Problems
Human papillomavirus (HPV)	Genital warts; cancers of the cervix, vulva, penis, and mouth/throat.
Chlamydia	Can lead to pelvic inflammatory disease and life-threatening ectopic pregnancy in women, as well as infertility; in pregnant women who become infected, fetus can develop severe health problems.
Gonorrhea	Can lead to pelvic inflammatory disease and life-threatening ectopic pregnancy in women, as well as infertility; can spread to the blood and joints and become a life-threatening illness; in pregnant women, fetus can develop severe health problems.
Syphilis	If disease progresses without treatment, damage can occur to the heart, blood vessels, liver, bones, and joints; advanced cases can affect the nerves, eyes, and brain, and can cause death; severe health risks for fetus in pregnant women.
Human immunodeficiency virus (HIV)	Can potentially destroy the human immune system, leaving the sufferer vulnerable to deadly infections and diseases; most advanced stage is known as AIDS.
Genital herpes	Painful, watery skin blisters on or around the genitals or anus; in pregnant women, fetus can develop a life-threatening illness known as neonatal HSV, which affects the skin, brain, and other organs.
Trichomoniasis	Especially dangerous for pregnant women; can cause premature birth and low birth weight; infants born to infected mothers are twice as likely to be stillborn or to die as newborns.
Viral hepatitis	Certain types can cause serious damage to the liver, which can lead to liver scarring (cirrhosis), cancer, liver failure, and death.

Source: National Institute of Child Health and Human Development, "What Are Some Types of STDs/STIs?," November 30, 2012. www.nichd.nih.gov.

Women Unaware of Trichomoniasis

The parasitic STD called trichomoniasis can be risky for women, causing everything from itching and burning in the vagina to increased risk of being infected with HIV. Yet according to a 2013 survey by the American Sexual Health Association, awareness of trichomoniasis is lower than for all other STDs.

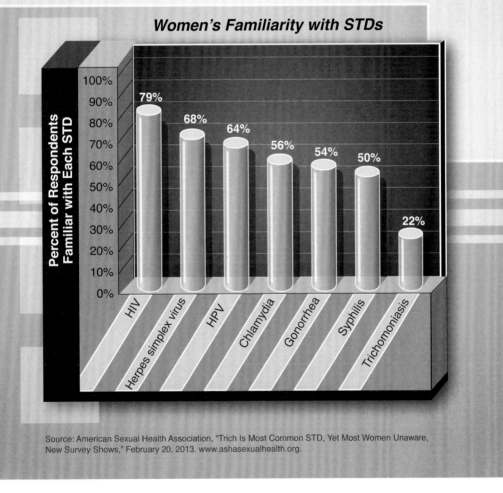

Women's Familiarity with STDs

Percent of Respondents Familiar with Each STD

- HIV: 79%
- Herpes simplex virus: 68%
- HPV: 64%
- Chlamydia: 56%
- Gonorrhea: 54%
- Syphilis: 50%
- Trichomoniasis: 22%

Source: American Sexual Health Association, "Trich Is Most Common STD, Yet Most Women Unaware, New Survey Shows," February 20, 2013. www.ashasexualhealth.org.

- According to the NICHD, **pregnant women** with trichomoniasis are twice as likely to have stillborn babies or babies that die soon after birth than are uninfected mothers.

How Can STDs Be Prevented?

❝Primary prevention of STDs begins with changing the sexual behaviors that place persons at risk for infection.❞

—Centers for Disease Control and Prevention, the United States' leading health protection agency.

❝The only 100 percent effective way to avoid an STI is not to have oral, vaginal or anal sex at all.❞

—Palo Alto Medical Foundation, a health care organization that serves the California counties of Alameda, San Mateo, Santa Clara, and Santa Cruz.

In February 2013, when the CDC released a report on STD prevalence in the United States, many health care professionals were shocked by the high numbers. The report showed that there were an estimated 110 million cases of STDs in the United States, with 20 million new infections each year. More than half of those new cases were adolescents and young adults. CDC epidemiologist Catherine Satterwhite was lead author of the report, and she speaks candidly about the urgency of prevention and treatment efforts. "All STIs are preventable," she says. "They're all treatable, and many are curable. But if they're left untreated, they can lead to pretty serious lifelong problems and even death."[54]

The Challenge of Changing Behaviors

Also in her statement, Satterwhite emphasizes the need for people to be aware of the risks involved with STDs and to take personal responsibility for protecting themselves. "Individuals need to talk openly to their sexual partners," she says, "and to their doctors about getting tested and they need to reduce their individual risk. They need to vaccinate. They need to consider ways to reduce their risk like practicing abstinence, using condoms correctly and consistently every time, and being in a mutually monogamous relationship."[55]

Few would disagree with Satterwhite's contention that preventing STDs is important—but it would be a task of epic proportions. Preventing STDs involves changing the behaviors of billions of people throughout the world. The immensity of this challenge was addressed by the Global HIV Prevention Working Group, a panel of public health experts, clinicians, biomedical and behavioral researchers, and advocates. Referring specifically to HIV, the report authors write: "Human behavior is complex; widespread behavior changes are challenging to achieve; and there are important gaps in our knowledge about the effectiveness of HIV prevention. Yet the research to date clearly documents the impact of numerous behavioral interventions in reducing HIV infection."[56]

Practicing Safer Sex

One behavioral change that infectious disease experts say is critical to curtailing STDs is consistent and correct use of latex condoms, as the CDC explains: "Inconsistent use can lead to STD acquisition because transmission can occur with a single act of intercourse with an infected partner. Similarly, if condoms are not used correctly, the protective effect may be diminished even when they are used consistently."[57] The CDC adds that latex condoms have proved to be highly effective in preventing HIV, as well as other STDs such as gonorrhea, chlamydia, and trichomoniasis.

The agency emphasizes, however, that even when condoms are used as recommended they provide "different levels of protection for various STDs." For instance, condoms can help protect against HPV and genital sores, or ulcers, caused by syphilis and genital herpes, but protection may be limited. "Latex condoms can only protect against transmission when the ulcers or infections are in genital areas that are covered or protected

> **Preventing STDs involves changing the behaviors of billions of people throughout the world.**

by the condom," says the CDC. "Thus, consistent and correct use of latex condoms would be expected to protect against transmission of genital ulcer diseases and HPV in some, but not all, instances."[58]

Evaluating the prevalence of condom use among high school students was one focus of a CDC report that examined young people's risk behaviors. Released in July 2012, the report contained both good news and bad news about condom use among teens: More of them are using condoms than twenty years ago, but the percentage of use has been declining since 2003. When teens were surveyed in 1991 about condom use the last time they had sex, 46.2 percent said that they had used a condom. By 2003 that number was up to 63 percent, but then it began to decline and was at 60.2 percent in 2011. Kevin Fenton, who directs the CDC's National Center for HIV/ AIDS, Viral Hepatitis, STD, and TB Prevention, says that the overall increase in condom use among teens since 1991 is "good news," but because of the decline since 2003, he adds: "We need to do a lot more."[59]

> **More [teens] are using condoms than twenty years ago, but the percentage of use has been declining since 2003.**

One-Click Condoms

In an effort to reduce the rate of STD transmission among teenagers in California, state health officials launched a program in February 2012. Known as the Condom Access Project (CAP), the program's focus is twofold: preventing STDs by expanding awareness of the importance of condom use, and making condoms easily accessible to young people. Says the Family Health Council's Amy Moy: "We can't keep our heads in the sand and pretend there isn't a problem. . . . We want to make sure (teens are) as safe as possible."[60] Once per month, anyone between the ages of twelve and nineteen in participating counties can go online and confidentially request a pack of ten condoms. The teens also receive educational information as well as personal lubricant to reduce the chance of condom breakage.

Not everyone is convinced that the program is a good one. In fact many are opposed, saying that young people could perceive that the state is encouraging them to have sex. This, critics say, is sure to evoke anger from parents, as Linda Davis, a spokeswoman for the Bakersfield Pregnancy Center in central California's Kern County, explains: "I would think the overwhelming majority of parents in Kern County wouldn't think this is a good idea. And I don't think their kids would have the nerve to request them."[61]

Underutilized Protection

Referring to the HPV vaccine as a "strong weapon to prevent several types of cancer in our kids,"[62] the CDC recommends that the vaccination be given to preteen girls and boys (aged eleven or twelve) before they become sexually active. There are two vaccines, which together prevent infection from high-risk strains of HPV. They protect against cervical, vulva, and vaginal cancers in women, as well as anal cancer and most cases of genital warts in both women and men.

According to a study released by the CDC in June 2013, the HPV vaccine is a true success story because it saves lives. CDC scientist Lauri Markowitz and her colleagues conducted the study using data from the National Health and Nutrition Examination Survey. They analyzed the prevalence of HPV infection among girls and women aged fourteen to fifty-nine from 2003 to 2006 (before the start of the HPV vaccination program) and compared it with prevalence after the vaccine became available (from 2007 to 2010). Published in the *Journal of Infectious Diseases*, the study reveals that since the vaccine was introduced, the prevalence of "vaccine-type" HPV infections decreased 56 percent among females aged fourteen to nineteen. "This decline is encouraging," says Markowitz, "given the substantial health and economic burden of HPV-associated disease."[63]

> " According to a study released by the CDC in June 2013, the HPV vaccine is a true success story because it saves lives. "

One month after that study was released, another CDC study was announced—but its findings were not promising. Researchers found that only slightly more than half of girls in the United States aged thirteen to seventeen had been given the HPV vaccination, and the number did not increase between 2011 and 2012. Among unvaccinated girls, 84 percent missed the opportunity to be vaccinated for HPV when they visited a health care provider for another immunization. The final report states that if the girls had received an HPV vaccine at that time, the rate of girls who were vaccinated with at least one dose could be as high as 93 percent.

Searching for Answers

To evaluate the reasons for the low HPV vaccination rates among girls, a team of researchers led by Oklahoma pediatrician Paul M. Darden conducted a study that was published in the medical journal *Pediatrics* in 2013. The team evaluated a three-year CDC survey of American families with thirteen- to seventeen-year-old children, that involved parents being asked a number of general questions about vaccinations. If the parents chose not to vaccinate, they were asked to share their reasons. The findings were discouraging, as the study authors write: "Despite doctors increasingly recommending adolescent vaccines, parents increasingly intend not to vaccinate female teens with HPV."[64]

The study revealed that over time, more parents were expressing that they had no plans to have their daughters vaccinated. Among parents whose daughters were not up-to-date on the HPV vaccine in 2008, 40 percent said they did not intend for their daughters to get this vaccine. By 2010 the number who gave that response had increased to 44 percent. The most perplexing finding of the study was inexplicable safety concerns about the vaccine. Between 2008 and 2010, the number of parents who cited safety as one reason their daughter had not been vaccinated nearly quadrupled. Although there have been reports of adverse effects of the vaccine, the CDC says those have never been confirmed as definitely linked to the vaccine. Also, there have been no recent reports, which is why the parents' rising safety concerns was such a surprise.

Sending the Wrong Message?

Since the HPV vaccine was first introduced, one of the biggest controversies was that it was implicitly encouraging teens to become sexually active. Of the groups that spoke out against it, none was more adamant in its opposition than the Family Research Council. Bridget Maher, the group's policy analyst on marriage and family, warned in 2006 that "giving the HPV vaccine to young women could be potentially harmful, because they may see it as a license to engage in premarital sex."[65]

To investigate the validity of this claim, a team of researchers conducted a study that was published in the medical journal *Pediatrics* in October 2012. It involved 1,398 girls, 493 of whom had been vaccinated for HPV and 905 who had not. After a comprehensive investigation to evaluate the girls' sexual activity (or lack thereof), the team found that there was no connection between the vaccine and sexual behavior. Referring to the study findings, New York adolescent medicine specialist Elizabeth Alderman says it will help her ease the minds of anxious parents: "I'll now be able to use this study as a piece of evidence to show them that it's not going to give girls a license to [engage in] sexual activity."[66]

Teens Helping Teens

Since 1997 MTV has partnered with the Kaiser Family Foundation on a public service campaign to help young people make responsible decisions about their sexual health. One of the focuses has been preventing the spread of HIV and other STDs through a program called "Get Yourself Tested" (GYT). As part of this effort, a new campaign was launched in November 2012 called "I'm Positive," which is a mini–reality show. It features three young people (Kelly, Stephanie, and Otis), all of whom are HIV positive and doing their best to cope with the challenges of living with the infection.

A key message of the GYT campaign is encouraging young people, whether they are HIV positive or not, to join in the fight against HIV and AIDS in the United States. Five core actions are emphasized: being informed; speaking out; using protection; getting tested; and, for those who are HIV positive, getting into care and staying on treatment. MTV has kept the conversation going by promoting it on Twitter, where it "is meant to ignite a dialogue around the role that young people can play in an AIDS free future."[67]

> [Twenty] million new cases of STDs are still reported each year in the United States alone, which is a strong indication that more needs to be done.

Kelly, a young woman from California, says that her participation in the MTV program is one of many ways that she is helping to prevent AIDS and HIV. Since Kelly learned that she was HIV positive, she has participated in the AIDS walk in Los Angeles, helped create a documentary for her school, and given ongoing presentations to young people. "I don't want anybody to experience getting diagnosed," she says. "If I can help one person avoid getting this disease by telling my story then I've done something great in the world." Kelly has lofty goals, as she explains: "I just want to help people. I want to change the world for the better—and I think I can do it."[68]

Immense Challenges

There are numerous ways that STDs can be prevented, but at the root of prevention is changing people's behaviors—and that is an enormous challenge. Efforts are under way to help educate people about STD prevention methods, including more widespread use of condoms and the importance of vaccines that help prevent infection by high-risk strains of HPV. Programs such as MTV's "Get Yourself Tested" help create awareness among young people about HIV and how infection can be prevented. These and other efforts are making a difference. But 20 million new cases of STDs are still reported each year in the United States alone, which is a strong indication that more needs to be done.

Primary Source Quotes*

How Can STDs Be Prevented?

66 Teenagers should be instructed on how to practice safe sex to avoid STIs. 99

—American Academy of Pediatrics, "Pelvic Inflammatory Disease," July 1, 2013. www.healthychildren.org.

The American Academy of Pediatrics is dedicated to the health, safety, and well-being of infants, children, adolescents, and young adults.

66 There really is no such thing as 'safe' sex. The only truly effective way to prevent STDs is abstinence. 99

—Melissa Conrad Stöppler, "Sexually Transmitted Diseases (STDs) in Women," MedicineNet, April 12, 2012. www.medicinenet.com.

Stöppler is a physician who serves on the medical editorial board of MedicineNet.com and is chief medical editor of eMedicineHealth.com.

Bracketed quotes indicate conflicting positions.

* Editor's Note: While the definition of a primary source can be narrowly or broadly defined, for the purposes of Compact Research, a primary source consists of: 1) results of original research presented by an organization or researcher; 2) eyewitness accounts of events, personal experience, or work experience; 3) first-person editorials offering pundits' opinions; 4) government officials presenting political plans and/or policies; 5) representatives of organizations presenting testimony or policy.

66 I like to use the term safer sex because I don't think that sex is ever entirely safe for lots of reasons, but condoms reduce the risk of transmission by about 50 percent. 99

—Peter Leone, "Even Without Symptoms, Genital Herpes Can Spread," NPR *Science Friday*, April 15, 2011. www.npr.org.

Leone is an infectious disease specialist at the University of North Carolina School of Medicine and medical director of the North Carolina HIV/STD Prevention and Control Branch.

66 No serious HPV vaccine side effects have been found, although fainting spells following injection have been reported in teens and young adults. 99

—WebMD, "HPV Vaccines," HPV/Genital Warts Health Center, August 13, 2012. www.webmd.com.

With content monitored by a staff of physicians, WebMD is one of the Internet's leading health information resources.

66 WebMD had the gall to misinform the public by stating that there have been NO serious side effects associated with HPV vaccination! What parent would not consider even the remote potential for permanent disability and/or death worthy of at least a brief mention? 99

—Joseph M. Mercola, "New Evidence Demolishes Claims of Safety and Effectiveness of HPV Vaccine," Mercola.com, October 16, 2012. http://articles.mercola.com.

Mercola is a physician who advocates alternative medicine and who is known for his strong views against conventional medical techniques and drugs.

66 Abstinence, monogamy, and consistent condom use are the primary HIV/STD-protective behaviors that public health intervention efforts target for adolescents and young adults. 99

—Ralph J. DiClemente, Jessica McDermott Sales, Fred Danner, and Richard A. Crosby, "Association Between Sexually Transmitted Disease and Young Adults' Self-Reported Abstinence," *Pediatrics*, January 3, 2011. http://pediatrics.aappublications.org.

DiClemente, Sales, Danner, and Crosby are medical researchers.

❝Some common STDs are curable, while others are incurable but treatable. All, however, are preventable.❞

—National Institute of Allergy and Infectious Diseases (NIAID), "STD Prevention Research: An International Effort," April 4, 2012. www.niaid.nih.gov.

The NIAID conducts and supports research to better understand, treat, and ultimately prevent infectious, immunologic, and allergic diseases.

❝STD prevention is an essential primary care strategy for improving reproductive health.❞

—US Department of Health and Human Services (HHS), "Sexually Transmitted Diseases," April 10, 2013. www.healthypeople.gov.

The HHS is the US government's principal agency for protecting the health of all Americans.

❝Increased public awareness and advancements in medicine over the past three decades have led to remarkable strides in preventing the spread of HIV.❞

—Office of Adolescent Health, "Teens and the HIV/AIDS Epidemic," June 2012. www.hhs.gov.

An agency of the US Department of Health and Human Services, the Office of Adolescent Health is committed to improving the health and well being of adolescents to enable them to become healthy, productive adults.

❝Preventing STDs is important for all sexually active individuals, but especially so for people living with HIV.❞

—Ronald Valdiserri, "STD Prevention, Screening, and Treatment Helps Prevent HIV Transmission and Ensure Health of People Living with HIV," *AIDS.gov* (blog), April 26, 2013. http://blog.aids.gov.

Valdiserri is deputy assistant secretary for health and infectious diseases and is director of the US Department of Health and Human Service Office of HIV/AIDS and Infectious Disease Policy.

Facts and Illustrations

How Can STDs Be Prevented?

- The CDC estimates that fewer than **half** of people who should be screened for STDs (such as sexually active youth aged fifteen to twenty-four and pregnant women) undergo recommended screening services.

- According to the American Congress of Obstetricians and Gynecologists, one way of preventing STDs is to avoid **anal sex**, as tissues in the rectum tear easily and can allow infectious organisms to get into the bloodstream.

- A 2013 study by researchers from the University of California at Los Angeles found that **Facebook and other social networking technologies** could serve as effective tools for preventing HIV infection among at-risk groups.

- According to the NICHD, AIDS can be prevented by early initiation of **antiretroviral therapy** in those who are infected with HIV.

- Infectious disease specialist Kimberly Workowski states that **STD screening**, combined with **treatment**, is one of the most effective tools available to protect people's health and prevent the spread of STDs.

- The World Health Organization states that universal screening and treatment for syphilis among pregnant women could prevent nearly a **half-million syphilis-related stillbirths** and newborn deaths in sub-Saharan Africa alone.

Risks Can Be Reduced

Although sexual abstinence is the only 100 percent reliable means of preventing STDs, the risk of contracting STDs can be greatly reduced through a variety of steps.

Stay with one partner	Remain in a long-term, mutually monogamous relationship with a partner who is not infected.
Get vaccinated	Vaccines can prevent two viral STDs: HPV and hepatitis A and B (HPV vaccine for girls/women through age twenty-six, and boys/men through age twenty-six).
Wait and verify	Vaginal and anal intercourse with new partners should be avoided until both have been tested.
Practice safe sex	A new latex condom or dental dam should be used for each sex act, whether oral, vaginal, or anal. Oil-based lubricants should be avoided.
Avoid excessive drinking or drugs	People under the influence are more likely to engage in risky sexual behavior.
Avoid anonymous, casual sex	Not knowing a sex partner increases the chances of exposure to an STD.
Communicate	Before any serious sexual contact, partners should talk about practicing safer sex and reach an explicit agreement about what activities will and will not be okay.
Consider male circumcision	Evidence has shown that male circumcision can reduce a man's risk of acquiring HIV from an infected woman by up to 60 percent.
Consider the drug Truvada	An FDA-approved drug that can help reduce the risk of contracting HIV in those who are considered at high risk for infection. Only appropriate for people who do not already have HIV or hepatitis B infection—and must be obtained through a doctor.

Source: Mayo Clinic, "Sexually Transmitted Diseases," February 23, 2013. www.mayoclinic.com.

- According to the Mayo Clinic, HPV screening is **only available for women** and not for men.

- The NIH says that one preventive step for women is to avoid having sex during **menstruation**, as they are more susceptible to catching STDs during that time.

Progress in Reducing Risky Teen Behavior

In July 2012 the Centers for Disease Control and Prevention reported on changes in the sexual habits of high school students between 1991 and 2011. In their study, the researchers found that fewer teens are having sex with multiple partners while at the same time more teens, in general, are using condoms.

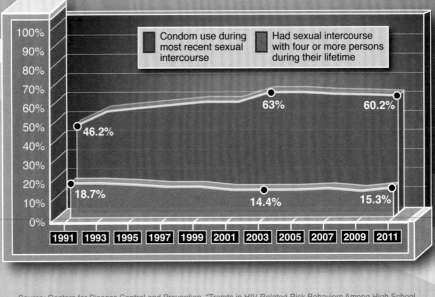

Source: Centers for Disease Control and Prevention, "Trends in HIV-Related Risk Behaviors Among High School Students—United States, 1991–2011," *Morbidity and Mortality Weekly Report*, July 27, 2012. www.cdc.gov.

- According to the CDC, **male circumcision** has been shown to reduce the risk of HIV transmission from women to men during vaginal sex.

- The World Health Organization states that the HPV vaccine could prevent the deaths of more than 4 million women over the next decade in low- and middle-income countries if **70 percent** vaccination coverage can be achieved.

Most Do Not Favor HPV Vaccine Without Parental Consent

Two HPV vaccines have been developed, which together protect against most cases of genital warts and several types of cancer. Most adults who participated in a 2012 University of Michigan survey are in favor of young people (aged twelve to seventeen) being able to access prevention and treatment of STDs without parental consent, which is already legal in all US states. In terms of the HPV vaccine, however, the majority of respondents believe that parental consent should be required.

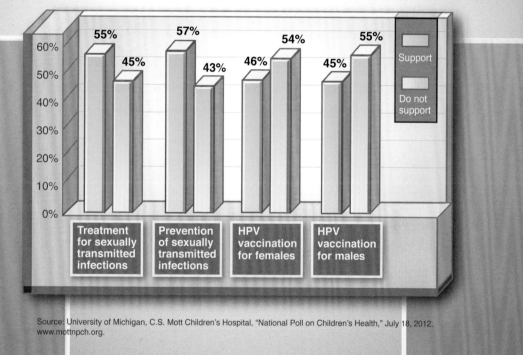

Adult Views on Teens Getting STD Care Without Parental Consent

Source: University of Michigan, C.S. Mott Children's Hospital, "National Poll on Children's Health," July 18, 2012. www.mottnpch.org.

- The Mayo Clinic states that the drug called **Truvada** can help reduce the risk of sexually transmitted HIV infection in those who are at high risk.

- According to the CDC, **latex condoms** are highly effective at preventing the transmission of HIV.

What Progress Has Been Made in the Fight Against STDs?

❝Despite their burdens, costs, and complications, and the fact that they are largely preventable, STDs remain a significant public health problem in the United States.❞

—US Department of Health and Human Services (HHS), the US government's principal agency for protecting the health of all Americans.

❝There are some STDs that respond to medication therapies, and with treatment, the symptoms associated with these disorders can be kept well in check. However, the diseases never really disappear altogether, meaning that the teen will have the disease for the rest of his/her life.❞

—Newport Academy, a Southern California teen treatment center.

When evaluating the extraordinary progress that has been made in the ongoing battle against STDs, health officials, infectious disease experts, and medical groups often use HIV as an example. Once considered a devastating and fatal infection, the virus no longer poses the threat it once did. The American Academy of Pediatrics writes: "For the first ten years of the AIDS crisis, the disease was a virtual death sentence for most of its victims. Few survived more than two years, on average. However, today there are many different types of medications available for the control of HIV. While HIV remains incurable, good adherence to medications can allow those infected to lead long productive lives and never develop AIDS."[69]

Paige Rawl, an eighteen-year-old woman from Indianapolis, Indiana, was born to a mother who was infected with HIV, and Rawl caught the virus before she was born. She is living proof that those who are HIV positive can live happy, healthy lives. In October 2013 the attractive blonde teenager appeared on the cover of *Seventeen* as one of five finalists for the magazine's "Pretty Amazing" contest. Rawl takes what is known as highly active antiretroviral therapy (HAART). It has resulted in the HIV in her bloodstream being suppressed to the point of being undetectable. In other words, even though the virus is present in her body, it does not attack her immune system.

This sort of progress is an enormous change from years ago before Rawl was born, as infectious disease specialist H. Reid Mattison explains: "In essence, it was 100 percent fatal. When you were diagnosed with HIV in the era prior to effective treatment, you knew eventually the virus was going to win in a matter of time."[70]

Hope for Babies

According to Michel Sidibé, the executive director of the organization UNAIDS, worldwide more than three hundred thousand infants are born HIV positive each year. Without proper medication—which is scarce to nonexistent in many poverty-stricken developing countries— most of these babies die before they are two years old. That bleak outlook is a major reason why a March 2013 announcement was met with such excitement on the part of many people who witnessed it.

At a medical conference in Atlanta, Georgia, a team of physicians announced that a child from Mississippi who was born HIV positive had been cured. Now two and a half years old, the little girl was started on a regimen of antiretroviral therapy within thirty hours of her birth. This involved a three-drug "cocktail" that was given to the baby every day for eighteen months. It was much stronger and administered more swiftly than is typical for HIV treatment. By the time the doctors made the 2013 announcement, the child had been off medication for over a year and is no longer infected. "This is a really groundbreaking report," says Diane Havlir, a professor and AIDS researcher at the University of California at San Francisco. "This tells us a cure is possible. That is thrilling news."[71]

The news about the Mississippi baby was hailed as an exciting step forward in the fight against HIV and AIDS. Health officials emphasize, however, that the priority should be preventing the babies from being born with the virus in the first place—and there has been extraordinary progress in accomplishing that. In June 2013 US Secretary of State John Kerry announced that 1 million HIV-free babies had been born to HIV-positive mothers, and thirteen countries are now at an AIDS "tipping point," meaning that more people are newly receiving treatment than are newly infected. Eric Goosby, who is the US global AIDS coordinator, says that pediatric intervention is crucial to stopping the spread of HIV, and that strides in treatment for pregnant women have been huge. This has resulted in far fewer babies being born with HIV.

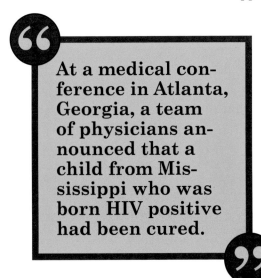

> At a medical conference in Atlanta, Georgia, a team of physicians announced that a child from Mississippi who was born HIV positive had been cured.

Germ Busters

Infectious disease experts say that people who suffer from bacterial or parasitic STDs can be more easily treated and cured because the conditions respond so well to antibiotics. Also known as antimicrobial drugs, antibiotics are medications that fight infections caused by certain types of pathogens, such as those that cause syphilis, gonorrhea, chlamydia, and trichomoniasis.

Over time, some pathogens that were formerly curable by antibiotics have become antibiotic-resistant. What this means is that bacteria are developing resistance to the drugs faster than new drugs can be developed. This creates a dangerous situation that the CDC refers to as "one of the world's most pressing public health problems," as the agency explains:

"Almost every type of bacteria has become stronger and less responsive to antibiotic treatment when it is really needed. These antibiotic-resistant bacteria can quickly spread to family members, schoolmates, and co-workers—threatening the community with a new strain of infectious disease that is more difficult to cure and more expensive to treat."[72]

Battling the "Superbug"

One of the STDs that scientists warn has become resistant to antibiotics is gonorrhea. In the past, the disease was easily cured with several types of antibiotic medications, but in July 2013 the CDC announced that this was no longer the case. The agency explains: "While antibiotics have long been successfully used to treat gonorrhea, the bacteria has eventually grown resistant to every drug ever used to treat it."[73] Based on these new findings, the CDC pared down its treatment recommendation for gonorrhea to include just one class of antibiotics that was still believed to be effective. But the CDC cited surveillance data and other evidence "that suggest it is only a matter of time before gonorrhea becomes resistant to the only remaining treatments currently available."[74] In news stories, this antibiotic-resistant strain of gonorrhea has been widely referred to as a "superbug."

A discovery announced in June 2013 by researchers at Boston University in Massachusetts may potentially solve the problem of antibiotic-resistant STDs and other diseases. The team, led by biomedical engineer James Collins, performed laboratory experiments with mice. After adding a small amount of silver to antibiotics, they found that the drugs became up to a thousand times more effective at fighting infection. An especially exciting finding was that the team used the silver-laced drugs against antibiotic-resistant strains of bacteria, and that proved to be effective as well—the bacteria lost their resistance.

> Over time, some pathogens that were formerly curable by antibiotics have become antibiotic-resistant.

Another potential solution to battling the superbug utilizes existing antibiotics that may not be effective separately, but are powerful enough to fight the bacteria when given in combination. A CDC study, whose findings were announced in July 2013, involved four hundred men and women aged fifteen to sixty who suffered from various types of untreated gonorrhea. One drug combination, which was given by injection, was found to be 100 percent effective at curing genital gonorrhea infection. The other combination, which was given in pill form, proved to be more than 99 percent effective. In people who suffered from gonorrhea infection in the throat or rectum, both regimens cured 100 percent of the infections.

The Promise of Stem Cells

Scientists have long known that human stem cells have immense potential for treating and curing innumerable injuries and illnesses. Stem cells are found throughout the body's tissues and organs at all stages of life, including before and after birth. Stem cells are unique cells because unlike ordinary cells (which have a specialized purpose, such as fighting infection or carrying oxygen through the blood), stem cells are unspecialized or "programmable." Thus, they have the chameleonlike ability to differentiate, or take on the characteristics of different cells in tissues and organs.

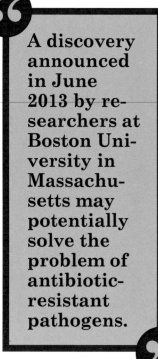

A discovery announced in June 2013 by researchers at Boston University in Massachusetts may potentially solve the problem of antibiotic-resistant pathogens.

In July 2013 researchers from Harvard Medical School and Brigham and Women's Hospital in Boston made an announcement about two HIV-positive patients who no longer have any sign of HIV in their bloodstreams. The patients, both men, had been on long-term antiretroviral therapy for their HIV infection when they developed lymphoma, which is cancer of the lymph nodes. To treat the cancer they both underwent chemotherapy, and then they each had a stem-cell transplant procedure. Eight months after the transplants were performed neither patient showed any sign of HIV. So, the researchers conducted a small clinical trial with the men. It involved withdrawing their antiretroviral therapy and performing ongoing blood analyses to watch for signs of the return of the virus in blood and other tissues. As of July 2013, neither patient showed evidence of any HIV in his blood. One had been off antiretroviral treatment for approximately fifteen weeks and the other for seven weeks.

Lead researcher Timothy Henrich says it is much too soon to draw any definitive long-term conclusions, and it would be premature to declare the patients cured of HIV. Still it is a finding with a great deal of promise. Kevin Robert Frost, who is chief executive of the Foundation for AIDS Research, shares his thoughts: "These findings clearly provide important new

> " There is no doubt that STDs are a serious problem in the United States and throughout the world, but medical science has achieved a great deal in terms of treating them. "

information that might well alter the current thinking about HIV and gene therapy. While stem-cell transplantation is not a viable option for people with HIV on a broad scale because of its costs and complexity, these new cases could lead us to new approaches to treating, and ultimately even eradicating, HIV."[75]

Clues Within T Cells

Herpes is one of the most frustrating STDs for sufferers because of the painful sores that develop in the genital areas. Says the CDC: "There can be considerable embarrassment, shame, and stigma associated with a herpes diagnosis and this can substantially interfere with a patient's relationships."[76] Unlike bacterial STDs, which can be cured with antibiotics, there is no cure for herpes, including the genital type. All antiviral medications can do is help keep outbreaks under control, and there is no guarantee that they will succeed in doing that.

An announcement in May 2013 may have offered people who suffer from genital herpes more hope than ever before. A team of scientists from Seattle's Fred Hutchinson Cancer Research Center and the University of Washington discovered a unique class of immune cells that are believed to be responsible for suppressing recurring outbreaks of genital herpes. The cells, known as CD8$\alpha\alpha$+ T cells, live in the genital skin and mucous membranes, and their identification could be the first step toward a possible cure for genital herpes or a vaccine to prevent it. Senior researcher Larry Corey explains: "If we can boost the effectiveness of these immune cells we are likely to be able to contain this infection at the point of attack and stop the virus from spreading in the first place. We're excited about our discoveries because these cells might also prevent other types of viral infections, including HIV infection."[77]

Hope for the Future

There is no doubt that STDs are a serious problem in the United States and throughout the world, but medical science has achieved a great deal in terms of treating them. HIV is no longer an automatic death sentence as it was in the 1980s, and STDs such as syphilis, chlamydia, and trichomoniasis can be completely cured. Antibiotic resistance is a distinct threat, but scientists are working hard to develop drugs that are capable of overcoming it. In the not-too-distant future, a vaccine or cure for genital herpes may become reality. As scientists continue to learn more about STDs in the coming years, treatments will undoubtedly become more sophisticated, and increasing numbers of infections may be cured. Hopefully these accomplishments will be significant enough to overcome the challenges.

What Progress Has Been Made in the Fight Against STDs?

> **The massive global expansion of access to HIV treatment has transformed not only the HIV epidemic but the entire public health landscape.**

—World Health Organization, *Global Update on HIV Treatment 2013: Results, Impact and Opportunities*, June 2013. http://apps.who.int.

The World Health Organization is the directing and coordinating authority for health within the United Nations system.

....

> **Although some STDs can be treated and cured, others cannot.**

—American Congress of Obstetricians and Gynecologists (ACOG), "How to Prevent Sexually Transmitted Diseases," May 2011. www.acog.org.

Composed of approximately fifty-five thousand physician members, the ACOG is the United States' leading advocate for women's quality health care.

....

* Editor's Note: While the definition of a primary source can be narrowly or broadly defined, for the purposes of Compact Research, a primary source consists of: 1) results of original research presented by an organization or researcher; 2) eyewitness accounts of events, personal experience, or work experience; 3) first-person editorials offering pundits' opinions; 4) government officials presenting political plans and/or policies; 5) representatives of organizations presenting testimony or policy.

❝As the lead agency for STD prevention in the United States, CDC will continue to improve both biomedical and behavioral strategies to combat STDs. Clearly, multiple strategies are required to maintain and improve progress.❞

—Centers for Disease Control and Prevention (CDC), "STD Prevention Today," National Prevention Information Network, April 12, 2013. www.cdcnpin.org.

The CDC is the United States' leading health protection agency.

❝While HIV/AIDS remains incurable, early diagnosis and treatment has allowed those who are HIV-infected to lead longer, productive lives.❞

—American Academy of Pediatrics, "Health Issues: Types of Sexually Transmitted Infections," July 1, 2013. www.healthychildren.org.

The American Academy of Pediatrics is dedicated to the health, safety, and well-being of infants, children, adolescents, and young adults.

❝Researchers at NCI and elsewhere are . . . studying what people know and understand about HPV and cancer, the best way to communicate to the public the latest research results, and how doctors are talking with their patients about HPV.❞

—National Cancer Institute (NCI), "Human Papillomavirus (HPV) Vaccines," NCI Fact Sheet, December 29, 2011. www.cancer.gov.

The NCI is the federal government's principal agency for cancer research and training.

❝While an HIV vaccine will be integral to achieving an AIDS-free generation, it also will be essential to realizing our ultimate goal: a world permanently without HIV/AIDS.❞

—Anthony S. Fauci, "An AIDS-Free Generation Is Closer than We Might Think," *Washington Post*, July 11, 2013.

Fauci is director of the National Institute of Allergy and Infectious Diseases.

66 Studies are underway to develop better treatments for the millions of people who suffer from genital herpes.**99**

—National Institute of Allergy and Infectious Diseases (NIAID), "Genital Herpes," January 6, 2012. www.niaid.nih.gov.

The NIAID conducts and supports research to better understand, treat, and ultimately prevent infectious, immunologic, and allergic diseases.

66 There is no cure for herpes, so the goals of treatment are to reduce the number of outbreaks and to lessen symptoms when you do have an outbreak.**99**

—University of Maryland Medical Center, "Herpes Simplex Virus," May 31, 2013. http://umm.edu.

The University of Maryland Medical Center is a teaching hospital in Baltimore that provides a full range of health services to people throughout Maryland and the mid-Atlantic region.

Facts and Illustrations

What Progress Has Been Made in the Fight Against STDs?

- According to a June 2013 report by the World Health Organization, **1.6 million** more people in low- and middle-income countries were receiving HIV treatment at the end of 2012 compared with the previous year, which represents the largest annual increase ever.

- The NIH says that advances in medicine have resulted in most STDs caused by bacteria and parasites to be **cured** if they are treated early enough.

- The CDC states that treatment for syphilis will kill the bacterium that causes the disease and prevent further health damage, but it will **not repair damage** that was already done.

- According to the Mayo Clinic, when people infected with HIV take their medications exactly as directed it is possible to **lower their virus** count to nearly undetectable levels.

- In a June 2013 report the World Health Organization states that the number of children younger than fifteen who are receiving HIV treatment rose from 566,000 in 2011 to **630,000** in 2012, but the percentage increase was smaller than for adults (**11 percent versus 21 percent**).

- According to the University of Maryland Medical Center, antiviral medicines can help shorten the length of a herpes outbreak and reduce the number of outbreaks by up to **80 percent**.

Many STDs Can Be Managed or Cured

Because of advances in medical science, bacterial and parasitic STDs can usually be cured with antibiotics. Those caused by viruses do not respond to antibiotics and are therefore incurable, although they can be managed with other types of medications. Shown here are treatments that are typically recommended for each STD.

STD	Type	Treatment
Chlamydia	Bacterial	Antibiotics
Gonorrhea	Bacterial	Antibiotics—Oral or injection
Syphilis	Bacterial	Antibiotics—Penicillin injection
Genital herpes	Viral	Antiviral medications to prevent frequent outbreaks
Hepatitis B	Viral	Difficult to treat; oral medications or injections are usually given
Human immunodeficiency virus (HIV)	Viral	Antiretroviral medications (combination of three or four) can slow progression of disease
Trichomoniasis	Parasitic	Antiparasitic and antibiotic medications

Source: Palo Alto Medical Foundation/Sutter Health, "Sexually Transmitted Infections—Treatment," 2013. www.pamf.org.

- The CDC states that antibiotics can successfully cure gonorrhea in adolescents and adults, but new **antibiotic-resistant strains** of the disease are increasing in many areas of the world.

- According to a December 2012 report by the group Cervical Cancer Action, cervical cancer rates in the United States continue to decline about **3 percent** each year, but comparable success has not been achieved in low- to middle-income countries.

Minors May Consent to STD Treatment Nationwide

All fifty US states have laws that give minors the authority to consent to health care, and this includes STD testing and treatment. As this map shows, some of the laws have contingencies, such as requiring that the minor be of a certain age and/or allowing physicians to notify parents that the minor is seeking/receiving services.

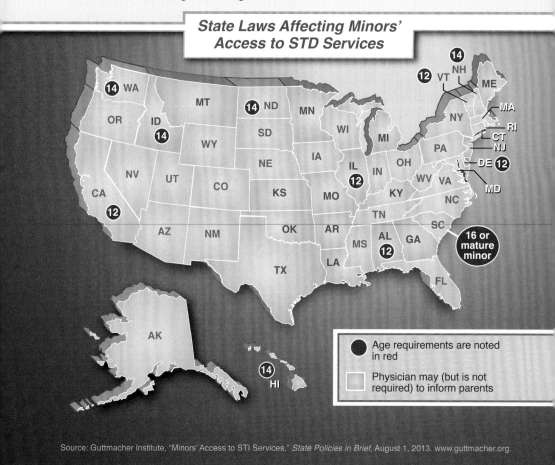

State Laws Affecting Minors' Access to STD Services

● Age requirements are noted in red

☐ Physician may (but is not required) to inform parents

16 or mature minor

Source: Guttmacher Institute, "Minors' Access to STI Services," *State Policies in Brief*, August 1, 2013. www.guttmacher.org.

- A 2013 document by the University of Maryland Medical Center cites a long-term study of fifty-three people with genital herpes, which found that those who were treated with **homeopathic therapies** (based on natural healing) experienced improvement in their symptoms and were less likely to have recurrent outbreaks.

AIDS Deaths Decline as Treatment Expands

HIV infection was once considered an automatic death sentence, but medical science has changed that prognosis drastically. Today millions of people who are HIV-positive are going about their lives, and their conditions may never even advance to the point of AIDS. This is largely due to antiretroviral therapy, which involves a combination of potent drugs. This graph shows how antiretroviral therapy has expanded throughout the world, with most of the expansion in sub-Saharan African countries where the need is greatest.

Number of people receiving antiretroviral therapy in low- and middle-income countries, by region, 2002—2011

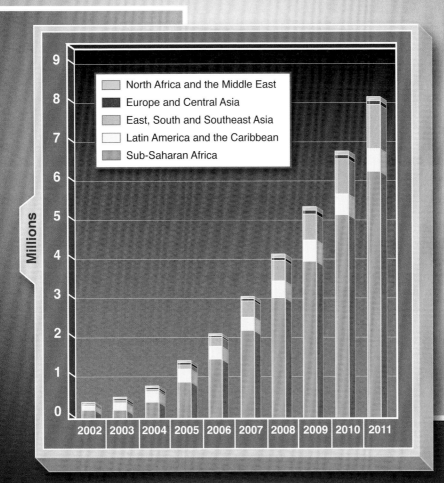

Source: UNAIDS, *Global Report*, November 20, 2012. www.unaids.org/en/media/unaids/contentassets/documents/ epidemiology/2012/gr2013/20121120_unaids_global_report_2012_with_annexes_en.pdf

Key People and Advocacy Groups

American Sexually Transmitted Diseases Association: A leading advocacy organization that is dedicated to the control and study of STDs.

Centers for Disease Control and Prevention (CDC): As the United States' leading health protection agency, the CDC is charged with promoting health and quality of life by controlling disease, injury, and disability.

Sir Alexander Fleming: A British scientist who in 1928 discovered the powerful antibiotic properties of the drug that he later called penicillin.

Foundation for AIDS Research: An organization dedicated to ending the global AIDS epidemic by supporting and helping to finance innovative research.

Robert Gallo: A scientist with the National Cancer Institute who linked HIV with AIDS and published his research in 1984 but was not credited for the discovery.

Beatrice H. Hahn: A researcher from the University of Alabama at Birmingham who led the international team of investigators in the discovery of HIV-1, the virus that leads to AIDS.

Ludwig Halberstaedter and Stanislaus von Prowazek: Czech scientists who in 1907 discovered the pathogenic bacterium that causes chlamydia.

Luc A. Montagnier and Françoise Barré-Sinoussi: French scientists who identified HIV, the virus that causes AIDS, and were awarded the Nobel Prize in Physiology or Medicine in 2008 for their discovery.

National Institute of Allergy and Infectious Diseases: An agency of the NIH that conducts and supports research to better understand, treat, and ultimately prevent infectious, immunologic, and allergic diseases.

Albert Ludwig Sigesmund Neisser: A German physician and bacteriologist who discovered gonococcus, the bacterium that causes gonorrhea, in 1879.

Georgios Papanicolaou: A scientist, originally from Greece, who is known for his cancer research and for the invention of the Pap smear, a diagnostic test for cervical cancer detection.

Planned Parenthood Federation of America: An organization that provides health care services, sex education, and sexual health information to women, men, and young people through its nearly nine hundred health centers throughout the United States.

Ernst Ruska: A German scientist who invented the electron microscope, which made it possible to observe viruses and other objects that are too tiny to be seen with ordinary microscopes.

Fritz Schaudinn and Erich Hoffmann: German scientists who in 1905 identified the pathogenic bacterium that causes syphilis.

Richard E. Shope: An American scientist who was the first to isolate the papilloma virus in cottontail rabbits and observe that the virus induced warts.

Harald zur Hausen: A German virologist who was the first to prove that the human papillomavirus (HPV) causes cervical cancer.

Chronology

1879
German physician and bacteriologist Albert Ludwig Sigesmund Neisser discovers gonococcus, the bacterium that causes gonorrhea.

1907
Working in Berlin, Germany, Czech scientists Ludwig Halberstaedter and Stanislaus von Prowazek discover the pathogenic bacterium that causes chlamydia.

1981
A report about a deadly type of pneumonia that primarily affects gay men appears in the CDC publication *Morbidity and Mortality Weekly Report*; this is later recognized as the first published scientific account of acquired immunodeficiency syndrome (AIDS).

1946
The Communicable Disease Center (CDC) opens in Atlanta, Georgia; years later its name is changed to the Centers for Disease Control and Prevention.

1930

1880

1980

1905
German researchers Fritz Schaudinn and Erich Hoffmann discover *Treponema pallidum*, the pathogenic bacterium that causes syphilis.

1933
American scientist Richard Shope becomes the first to isolate the papilloma virus in cottontail rabbits, and to observe that the virus induces warts.

1928
British scientist Sir Alexander Fleming notices that mold in a laboratory Petri dish has killed bacteria that were growing in the dish; by chance, Fleming has discovered the powerful antibiotic properties of what he later calls penicillin.

1970
Using an electron microscope, scientists J.D. Oriel and June Almeida discover virus particles in human genital warts and publish a paper about their findings in the *British Journal of Venereal Diseases*.

1974
At an international conference, German virologist Harald zur Hausen announces that the papilloma virus is the most significant cause of cervical cancer; his theory is rejected by his fellow scientists, and years go by before he is proved to be correct.

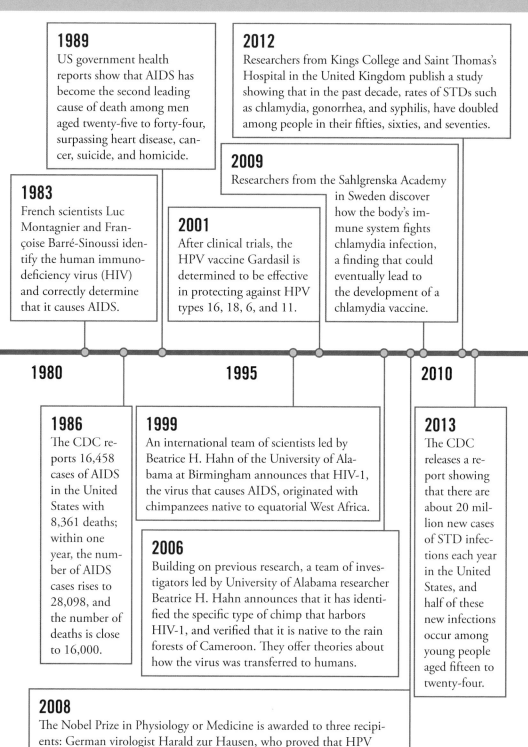

1989
US government health reports show that AIDS has become the second leading cause of death among men aged twenty-five to forty-four, surpassing heart disease, cancer, suicide, and homicide.

2012
Researchers from Kings College and Saint Thomas's Hospital in the United Kingdom publish a study showing that in the past decade, rates of STDs such as chlamydia, gonorrhea, and syphilis, have doubled among people in their fifties, sixties, and seventies.

2009
Researchers from the Sahlgrenska Academy in Sweden discover how the body's immune system fights chlamydia infection, a finding that could eventually lead to the development of a chlamydia vaccine.

1983
French scientists Luc Montagnier and Françoise Barré-Sinoussi identify the human immunodeficiency virus (HIV) and correctly determine that it causes AIDS.

2001
After clinical trials, the HPV vaccine Gardasil is determined to be effective in protecting against HPV types 16, 18, 6, and 11.

1980

1995

2010

1986
The CDC reports 16,458 cases of AIDS in the United States with 8,361 deaths; within one year, the number of AIDS cases rises to 28,098, and the number of deaths is close to 16,000.

1999
An international team of scientists led by Beatrice H. Hahn of the University of Alabama at Birmingham announces that HIV-1, the virus that causes AIDS, originated with chimpanzees native to equatorial West Africa.

2013
The CDC releases a report showing that there are about 20 million new cases of STD infections each year in the United States, and half of these new infections occur among young people aged fifteen to twenty-four.

2006
Building on previous research, a team of investigators led by University of Alabama researcher Beatrice H. Hahn announces that it has identified the specific type of chimp that harbors HIV-1, and verified that it is native to the rain forests of Cameroon. They offer theories about how the virus was transferred to humans.

2008
The Nobel Prize in Physiology or Medicine is awarded to three recipients: German virologist Harald zur Hausen, who proved that HPV causes cervical cancer, and French scientists Françoise Barré-Sinoussi and Luc Montagnier, who discovered HIV and proved that it causes AIDS.

Related Organizations

American Cancer Society

National Headquarters
250 Williams St.
Atlanta, GA 30303
phone: (404) 320-3333; toll-free: (800) 227-2345
website: www.cancer.org

The American Cancer Society is a nationwide, community-based voluntary health organization that is dedicated to eliminating cancer as a major health problem. Its website search engine produces a number of articles about STDs and their association with cancer.

American Congress of Obstetricians and Gynecologists (ACOG)

409 Twelfth St. SW
PO Box 70620
Washington, DC 20024-2188
phone: (202) 638-5577; toll-free: (800) 673-8444
website: www.acog.org

With more than fifty thousand members, ACOG serves as an advocate for quality health care for women. Its website provides a number of articles and fact sheets about STDs.

American Sexually Transmitted Diseases Association

PO Box 12665
Research Triangle Park, NC 27709
phone: (919) 861-9399
e-mail: astda@astda.org • website: www.astda.org

The American Sexually Transmitted Diseases Association is dedicated to the control and study of STDs. Its website offers news releases and links to a variety of resources, including newsletters, journals, and other related organizations.

Related Organizations

American Sexual Health Association

PO Box 13827
Research Triangle Park, NC 27709
phone: (919) 361-8400 • fax: (919) 361-8425
e-mail: info@ashastd.org • website: www.ashastd.org

The American Sexual Health Association serves as a source of reliable information on sexual health and STDs. Its website offers a great deal of information about STDs, including news releases, fact sheets, and reports, along with a link to the organization's blog.

Centers for Disease Control and Prevention (CDC)

1600 Clifton Rd.
Atlanta, GA 30333
phone: (404) 498-1515; toll-free: (800) 311-3435 • fax: (800) 553-6323
e-mail: inquiry@cdc.gov • website: www.cdc.gov/std

As the leading health protection agency in the United States, the CDC is charged with promoting health and quality of life by controlling disease, injury, and disability. Its STD website offers a wealth of information about STDs, including the various types, pathogens that cause them, risk factors, prevention, and treatment.

Foundation for AIDS Research

120 Wall St., 13th Floor
New York, NY 10005-3908
phone: (212) 806-1600 • fax: (212) 806-1601
website: www.amfar.org

The Foundation for AIDS Research is dedicated to ending the global AIDS epidemic by supporting and helping to finance innovative research. Its website provides a number of news articles and miscellaneous publications about HIV and its connection with AIDS.

Mayo Clinic

200 First St. SW
Rochester, MN 55905
phone: (800) 430-9699 • fax: (507) 284-0161
website: www.mayoclinic.com

Mayo Clinic is a nonprofit worldwide leader in medical care, research, and education. Its website search engine produces numerous publications about STDs.

National Institute of Allergy and Infectious Diseases (NIAID)

Office of Communications and Government Relations
6610 Rockledge Dr., MSC 6612
Bethesda, MD 20892-6612
phone: (301) 496-5717; toll-free: (866) 284-4107 • fax: (301) 402-3573
e-mail: ocpostoffice@niaid.nih.gov • website: www.niaid.nih.gov

An agency of the NIH, the NIAID conducts and supports research to better understand, treat, and ultimately prevent infectious, immunologic, and allergic diseases. Its website offers a variety of informative publications about STDs.

Planned Parenthood Federation of America

434 W. Thirty-Third St.
New York, NY 10001
phone: (212) 541-7800; toll free: (800) 230-7526 • fax: (212) 245-1845
website: www.plannedparenthood.org

Through its network of affiliates that operate nearly nine hundred health centers, Planned Parenthood provides health care services, sex education, and sexual health information to women, men, and young people. The search engine on its website produces numerous articles about the various types of STDs as well as risks, treatments, and prevention.

The STD Project

phone: (866) 944-1910
website: www.thestdproject.com

The STD Project is a progressive movement aimed at eradicating the stigmas around STDs by facilitating and encouraging awareness, education, and acceptance. A wealth of information can be found on its website, including news articles, fact sheets, and statistics, as well as links to blogs (separated by topic) and an online discussion forum.

World Health Organization

Avenue Appia 20
CH-1211 Geneva 27
Switzerland
phone: (41) 22 791 21 11 • fax: (41) 22 791 31 11
www.who.int

The World Health Organization is the directing and coordinating authority for health within the United Nations system. The search engine on its website produces numerous publications about STD types, risk factors, treatment challenges, prevention, and global trends.

For Further Research

Books

Nicholas Collins and Samuel G. Woods, *Frequently Asked Questions About STDs*. New York: Rosen, 2012.

H. Hunter Handsfield, *Color Atlas and Synopsis of Sexually Transmitted Diseases*. New York: McGraw-Hill, 2011.

Karen E. Rogstad, ed., *ABC of Sexually Transmitted Infections*. Chichester, West Sussex, UK: BMJ, 2011.

Lawrence R. Stanberry and Susan L. Rosenthal, *Sexually Transmitted Diseases: Vaccines, Prevention, and Control*. London: Academic Press, 2013.

Diane Yancey, *STDs*. Minneapolis, MN: Twenty-First Century, 2012.

Jonathan M. Zenilman and Mohsen Shahmanesh, eds., *Sexually Transmitted Infections: Diagnosis, Management, and Treatment*. Sudbury, MA: Jones & Bartlett, 2012.

Periodicals

Anthony S. Fauci, "An AIDS-Free Generation Is Closer than We Might Think," *Washington Post*, July 11, 2013.

Marissa Fessenden, "Yes, a Child Has Been Pronounced Cured of HIV—but Can It Be Duplicated?," *Scientific American*, March 5, 2013.

Denise Grady, "Troubles with Heart Are Linked to HPV," *New York Times*, October 24, 2011.

Jerome Groopman, "Sex and the Superbug," *New Yorker*, October 1, 2012.

Richa Gulati, "What You Need to Know About STDs," *Teen Vogue*, November 2012.

Anahad O'Connor, "Throat Cancer Link to Oral Sex Gains Notice," *New York Times*, June 3, 2013.

Mike Stobbe, "HPV Vaccine Cut Infection by Half in Teen Girls, Report Says," *Washington Post*, June 19, 2013.

Rachel Walden, "What You Need to Know About the HPV Vaccine," *Women's Health Activist*, July/August 2013.

Kurt Williamson, "The High Cost of 'Hooking Up,'" *New American*, January 7, 2013.

Internet Sources

Centers for Disease Control and Prevention, "STDs Today," National Prevention Information Network, April 16, 2013. www.cdcnpin .org/scripts/std/std.asp.

Centers for Disease Control and Prevention, "Sexually Transmitted Diseases: STDs & Pregnancy," CDC Fact Sheet, July 10, 2013. www .cdc.gov/std/pregnancy/stdfact-pregnancy.htm.

GirlsHealth.gov, "Body: Types of STIs," January 31, 2013. www.girls health.gov/body/sexuality/symptoms.html.

Healthline, "The 16 Best HIV/STD Health Blogs of 2013," June 26, 2013. www.healthline.com/health-slideshow/best-hiv-std-blogs.

Raychelle Cassada Lohmann, "STDs and Young People," *Psychology Today*, April 23, 2012. www.psychologytoday.com/blog/teen-angst/201204 /stds-and-young-people-0.

Meghan Neal, "Gonorrhea Superbug: First Antibiotic-Resistant STD Strain Discovered," *Huffington Post*, September 10, 2011. www.huff ingtonpost.com/2011/07/11/gonorrhea-superbug-antibiotic-resistant _n_894538.html.

Tara Parker-Pope, "HPV Vaccine Doesn't Alter Sexual Behavior, Study Finds," *New York Times*, October 15, 2012. Well (blog), http://well. blogs.nytimes.com.

Robert Preidt, "New Treatments Show Promise Against Drug-Resistant Gonorrhea," HealthDay, July 15, 2013. www.nlm.nih.gov/medline plus/news/fullstory_138716.html.

Peter A. Ubel, "Why James Bond Needs to Use Condoms," *Psychology Today, Scientocracy*, (blog), March 14, 2013. www.psychologytoday.com /blog/scientocracy/201303/why-james-bond-needs-use-condoms.

Urology Care Foundation, "Sexually Transmitted Infections (STIs)," March 2013. www.urologyhealth.org/urology/index.cfm?article=62.

Source Notes

Overview

1. Centers for Disease Control and Prevention, "Genital HPV Infection," July 25, 2013. www.cdc.gov.
2. Anonymous, "Girl Talk: I've Got an STD," *Clutch*, June 25, 2013. www.clutchmagon line.com.
3. Mayo Clinic, "Germs: Understand and Protect Against Bacteria, Viruses and Infection," April 30, 2011. www.mayoclinic.com.
4. James M. Steckelberg, "What's the Difference Between a Bacterial Infection and a Viral Infection?," Mayo Clinic: "Infectious Diseases," October 8, 2011. www.mayoclinic.com.
5. National Institutes of Health, "X-Plain: Sexually Transmitted Diseases," US National Library of Medicine, December 15, 2010. www.nlm.nih.gov.
6. American Sexual Health Association, "STDs/STIs," 2013. www.ashasexualhealth.org.
7. Yale Medical Group, "What You Need to Know about STDs," 2013. www.yalemedicalgroup.org.
8. American Congress of Obstetricians and Gynecologists, "How to Prevent Sexually Transmitted Diseases," May 2011. www.acog.org.
9. Student Health Services, "Sexually Transmitted Diseases (STDs)," University of North Carolina, Greensboro. http://shs.uncg.edu.
10. Henry J. Kaiser Family Foundation, *The HIV/AIDS Epidemic in the United States*, March 22, 2013. http://kff.org.
11. Centers for Disease Control and Prevention, "Parasites—Lice—Pubic 'Crab' Lice," November 2, 2010. www.cdc.gov.
12. Centers for Disease Control and Prevention, "Syphilis," CDC Fact Sheet, February 11, 2013. www.cdc.gov.
13. Amber, "My Name Is Amber," The Naked Truth, Idaho Department of Health & Welfare, July 2, 2012. www.nakedtruth.idaho.gov.
14. Mayo Clinic, "Sexually Transmitted Diseases (STDs)," February 23, 2013. www.mayoclinic.com.
15. Sara, "I Wish I Had Gone to the Doctor," The Naked Truth, Idaho Department of Health & Welfare, July 2, 2012. www.nakedtruth.idaho.gov.
16. Kimberly Workowski, *Sexually Transmitted Diseases: Office Management*, University of Utah School of Medicine, 2011. http://medicine.utah.edu.
17. Centers for Disease Control and Prevention, "STDs Today," National Prevention Information Network, April 16, 2013. www.cdcnpin.org.
18. National Institute of Child Health and Human Development, "What Are Some Types of STDs/STIs?," May 28, 2013. www.nichd.nih.gov.
19. National Institutes of Health, "X-Plain: Sexually Transmitted Diseases; Reference Summary," December 15, 2010. www.nlm.nih.gov.
20. Rima Himelstein, "Trich: This Sexually-Transmitted Disease Is No Treat," *Healthy Kids* blog, Philly.com, October 23, 2012. www.philly.com.
21. Mayo Clinic, "Sexually Transmitted Diseases (STDs)."
22. National Institute of Child Health and Human Development, "What Are the Treatments for STDs/STIs?," May 28, 2013. www.nichd.nih.gov.

23. Centers for Disease Control and Prevention, "Trichomoniasis—CDC Fact Sheet," August 3, 2012. www.cdc.gov.

What Are STDs?

24. Institute of Human Virology Jacques Initiative, "History of HIV/AIDS in the U.S." www.jacques.umaryland.edu.
25. Centers for Disease Control and Prevention, "Basic Information About HIV and AIDS," April 11, 2012. www.cdc.gov.
26. Kelly, "Kelly's Story," *I'm Positive*, MTV, November 26, 2012. www.mtv.com.
27. Kelly, "Kelly's Story."
28. Kaiser Family Foundation, *Sexual Health of Adolescents and Young Adults in the United States*, March 28, 2013. http://kff.org.
29. Harry Fisch, "Chlamydia," Men's Health. www.drharryfisch.com.
30. Quoted in Meghan E. Irons, "Chlamydia Targeted in Bowdoin-Geneva," *Boston Globe*, February 25, 2013. www.bostonglobe.com.
31. Quoted in Irons, "Chlamydia Targeted in Bowdoin-Geneva."
32. Peter Leone, "Even Without Symptoms, Genital Herpes Can Spread," NPR *Science Friday*, April 15, 2011. www.npr.org.
33. Leone, "Even Without Symptoms, Genital Herpes Can Spread."
34. Leone, "Even Without Symptoms, Genital Herpes Can Spread."
35. Victor, "I Found Out the Hard Way," The Naked Truth, Idaho Department of Health & Welfare, July 2, 2012. www.nakedtruth.idaho.gov.
36. Quoted in Frederik Joelving, "Viagra-Popping Seniors Lead the Pack for STDs," Reuters, July 6, 2010. www.webmd.com.
37. Quoted in Marni Jameson, "Seniors' Sex Lives Are Up—and So Are STD Cases Around the Country," *Orlando (FL) Sentinel*, April 18, 2011. http://articles.orlandosentinel.com.

What Are the Dangers of STDs?

38. Quoted in Emma Hooper, "'My Boyfriend Made Me Infertile,'" *River Online*, October 12, 2011. www.riveronline.co.uk.
39. Centers for Disease Control and Prevention, "Pelvic Inflammatory Disease (PID)," CDC Fact Sheet, September 28, 2011. www.cdc.gov.
40. Centers for Disease Control and Prevention, "Pelvic Inflammatory Disease (PID)."
41. Quoted in University of Edinburgh, "Chlamydia and Ectopic Pregnancy Link," January 24, 2011. www.ed.ac.uk.
42. Quoted in *Science Daily*, "Mechanism Leading from Trichomoniasis to Prostate Cancer Identified," August 30, 2012. www.sciencedaily.com.
43. Quoted in Theresa Tamkins, "Prostate Cancer Linked to Sexually Transmitted Disease," CNN, September 11, 2009. www.cnn.com.
44. National Cancer Institute, "HPV and Cancer," March 15, 2012. www.cancer.gov.
45. Rose Hansen, "'Common but Not Normal,': My HPV Positive Nightmare," *In Hue*, January 30, 2013. www.inhuemag.com/2013/01/30/common-but-not-normal-hpv.
46. Quoted in Hansen, "'Common but Not Normal,': My HPV Positive Nightmare."
47. Hansen, "'Common but Not Normal,': My HPV Positive Nightmare."
48. Hansen, "'Common but Not Normal,': My HPV Positive Nightmare."
49. Anil K. Chaturvedi et al. "Human Papillomavirus and Rising Oropharyngeal Cancer Incidence in the United States," *Journal of Clinical Oncology*, November 10, 2011. www.oralcancerfoundation.org.

50. Quoted in Xan Brooks, "Michael Douglas on Liberace, Cannes, Cancer and Cunnilingus," *Guardian*, June 2, 2013. www.theguardian.com.
51. Children's Hospital Colorado, "Immune System," October 2012. www.childrenscolorado.org.
52. Global Fund, Access to Life, "Questions and Answers." www.theglobalfund.org.
53. Global Fund, Access to Life, "Questions and Answers."

How Can STDs Be Prevented?

54. Quoted in Sanjay Gupta, "CDC: 20 Million New Sexually Transmitted Infections Yearly," CNN, February 13, 2013. http://thechart.blogs.cnn.com.
55. Quoted in Gupta, "CDC: 20 Million New Sexually Transmitted Infections Yearly."
56. Global HIV Prevention Working Group, *Behavior Change and HIV Prevention*, August 2008. www.globalhivprevention.org.
57. Centers for Disease Control and Prevention, "Condoms and STDs: Fact Sheet for Public Health Personnel," March 25, 2013. www.cdc.gov.
58. Centers for Disease Control and Prevention, "Condoms and STDs: Fact Sheet for Public Health Personnel."
59. Quoted in Fox News, "Researchers Report More Condom Use Among Teenagers," July 24, 2012. www.foxnews.com.
60. Quoted in Fox News, "California Counties Get Federally-Funded Teen Mail-Order Condom Program," February 19, 2012. www.foxnews.com.
61. Quoted in Thaddeus Baklinski, "California Govt. Mailing Condoms to Teenagers at Home in Unmarked Envelopes," *LifeSite News*, February 27, 2012. www.lifesitenews.com.
62. Centers for Disease Control and Prevention, "Diseases and the Vaccines That Prevent Them: HPV," July 2013. www.cdc.gov.
63. Quoted in Centers for Disease Control and Prevention, "New Study Shows HPV Vaccine Helping Lower HPV Infection Rates in Teen Girls," media release, June 19, 2013. www.cdc.gov.
64. Paul M. Darden et al. "Reasons for Not Vaccinating Adolescents: National Immunization Survey of Teens, 2008–2010," *Pediatrics*, March 18, 2013. http://pediatrics.aappublications.org.
65. Quoted in Nancy Gibbs, "Defusing the War Over the 'Promiscuity Vaccine,'" *Time*, June 21, 2006. www.time.com.
66. Quoted in Anahad O'Connor, "HPV Vaccine Doesn't Alter Sexual Behavior, Study Finds," *Well* (blog), *New York Times*, October 15, 2012. http://well.blogs.nytimes.com.
67. MTV, "MTV and Dr. Drew Team Up to Document the Lives of Three HIV Positive Young People in 'I'm Positive,' Premiering on World AIDS Day," press release, November 19, 2012. http://mtvpress.com.
68. Kelly, "Kelly's Story."

What Progress Has Been Made in the Fight Against STDs?

69. American Academy of Pediatrics, "Health Issues: Types of Sexually Transmitted Infections," HealthyChildren, July 1, 2013. www.healthychildren.org.
70. Quoted in Clara Ritger, "Teen Hopes Her Story of Living with HIV Helps Others," *USA Today*, June 22, 2013. www.usatoday.com.
71. Quoted in Liz Szabo, "Child's HIV Cure Won't Mean New Treatments Immediately," *USA Today*, March 4, 2013. www.usatoday.com.

72. Centers for Disease Control and Prevention, "Get Smart: Know When Antibiotics Work," July 9, 2013. www.cdc.gov/getsmart.

73. Centers for Disease Control and Prevention, "Gonorrhea Treatment Guidelines," CDC Fact Sheet, July 2013. www.cdc.gov.

74. Centers for Disease Control and Prevention, "Gonorrhea Treatment Guidelines."

75. Quoted in Foundation for AIDS Research, "Researcher Reports Two HIV Patients Showing No Signs of Virus in Wake of Stem-Cell Transplants," July 3, 2013. www.amfar.org.

76. Centers for Disease Control and Prevention, "Genital Herpes," CDC Fact Sheet, February 13, 2013. www.cdc.gov.

77. Quoted in Fred Hutchinson Cancer Research Center, "Immune Cells That Suppress Genital Herpes Infections Identified," May 8, 2013. www.fhcrc.org.

List of Illustrations

List of Illustrations

Index

Note: Boldface page numbers indicate illustrations.

Index

About the Author

Peggy J. Parks holds a bachelor of science degree from Aquinas College in Grand Rapids, Michigan, where she graduated magna cum laude. An author who has written more than a hundred educational books for children and young adults, Parks lives in Muskegon, Michigan, a town that she says inspires her writing because of its location on the shores of Lake Michigan.